P9-DNT-557

Cavewomen
Don't Get
Fat

Cavewomen Don't Get Fat

**THE PALEO CHIC DIET FOR
RAPID RESULTS**

Esther Blum, MS, RD, CDN, CNS

G

GALLERY BOOKS
New York   London   Toronto   Sydney   New Delhi

G

Gallery Books
A Division of Simon & Schuster, Inc.
1230 Avenue of the Americas
New York, NY 10020

First Gallery Books hardcover edition December 2013

GALLERY BOOKS and colophon are registered trademarks of Simon & Schuster, Inc.

For information about special discounts for bulk purchases, please contact Simon & Schuster Special Sales at 1-866-506-1949 or business@simonandschuster.com.

The Simon & Schuster Speakers Bureau can bring authors to your live event. For more information or to book an event contact the Simon & Schuster Speakers Bureau at 1-866-248-3049 or visit our website at www.simonspeakers.com.

Designed by Kyoko Watanabe

Manufactured in the United States of America

10 9 8 7 6 5 4 3 2 1

Library of Congress Cataloging-in-Publication Data

Blum, Esther.
Cavewomen don't get fat : the paleo chic diet for rapid results / Esther Blum MS, RD, CDN, CNS.
pages cm
Includes bibliographical references and index.
1. High-protein diet—Recipes. 2. Reducing diets—Recipes.
3. Prehistoric peoples—Nutrition. 4. Women—Nutrition. I. Title.
II. Title: Cavewomen don't get fat.
RM237.86.B58 2013
613.2'82—dc23 2013026431

ISBN 978-1-4767-0769-3
ISBN 978-1-4767-0771-6 (ebook)

Note to Readers

This publication contains the opinions and ideas of its author. It is intended to provide helpful and informative material on the subjects addressed in the publication. It is sold with the understanding that the author and publisher are not engaged in rendering medical, health, or any other kind of personal professional services in the book. The reader should consult his or her medical, health, or other competent professional before adopting any of the suggestions in this book or drawing inferences from it.

The author and publisher specifically disclaim all responsibility for any liability, loss, or risk, personal or otherwise, which is incurred as a consequence, directly or indirectly, of the use and application of any of the contents of this book.

For my parents, Florence and Larry,
with gratitude and love for a lifetime of support.

Contents

PART 1

Gorgeous Girls Gone Wild

PART 2

Modern Myths and Paleo Makeovers

PART 3

Cavewomen Don't Get Fat

Foreword

JJ VIRGIN, *NEW YORK TIMES* BESTSELLING
AUTHOR, *THE VIRGIN DIET*

Like you, I'm a busy woman juggling career and family, so I outsource some chores and responsibilities in order to focus on other things. But one thing I still do myself is grocery shop. I love wandering the aisles to see what new foods manufacturers impose on vulnerable consumers. Occasionally I am impressed, but far more often I'm dismayed at the fortified Frankenfoods and otherwise bizarre concoctions that pass for sustenance these days.

I can understand why people feel so confused about what they eat. Whole grain bread, which manufacturers tout as healthy, often contains high-fructose corn syrup (HFCS). Vitamin-fortified muffins, fiber-enriched cookies, and agave-sweetened soy ice cream create a halo effect, making you think that you're eating something healthy, when in reality you are eating junk food in disguise. And don't get me started about gluten-free cupcakes!

I often lament how far we've gotten from eating real food. So when Esther Blum told me about her back-to-basics approach in *Cavewomen Don't Get Fat*, I felt relieved to finally have a smart, savvy plan that simplifies the what-to-eat hype and hoopla.

Esther's Paleo Chic philosophy focuses on whole, unprocessed foods. This is the stuff that your great, great, great, great-grand-parents thrived on and your ancestors (I'm talking *thousands* of years ago) flourished on to stay trim, muscular, and healthy. After all, you had to be pretty lithe and lean in the cavewomen era, or you could end up a saber-toothed tiger's lunch!

When you eat foods that are lean and clean, there's little need to scrutinize labels or decipher ingredients. You know that no gluten (a protein found in wheat and other grains) slipped into your or-ganic broccoli and that your wild-caught salmon isn't injected with unpronounceable preservatives.

Esther uses her impressive scientific knowledge and training, coupled with years of experience counseling women on living gorgeously in Manhattan's concrete jungle, to bust some egregious "modern" dietary myths.

Hands up, for instance, if you've ever foolishly and drastically cut your calories to look like the latest skinny magazine cover model, who actually happens to be TOFI (thin on the outside, fat on the inside), but you ended up hungrier, grouchier, and flabbier after six weeks of starving yourself.

Esther shows you a smarter, healthier path toward burning fat, feeling your best, and turning back the clock that doesn't involve counting calories or any other calculations that take the fun out of eating.

What makes *Cavewomen Don't Get Fat* unique is that Esther goes beyond doling out diet advice to deliver cutting-edge tips that help you stay fit and fabulous, balance hormones, and detox-ify effectively. For instance, she debunks and explains why those store-bought tabloid-celebrity cleanses often do more harm than good.

Exercise is a vital part of the cavewoman protocol, but you probably don't have time for spin classes and elliptical machines amid your ever-growing to-do list. Thankfully, Esther shows you how to get that lean, mean cavewoman physique without spending hours in the gym.

Reduce stress? Get optimal shut-eye? Count me in. Esther's got smart strategies for that too.

Lest I make her sound overly serious and studious, Esther is *not* all work and no play. She's my favorite party girl nutritionist who can make science fun and sexy (*not* an easy thing to do!), and she shows you how to have a good time and keep your dietary dignity with no lingering regrets. There's even a section all about the power of chocolate. Enough said!

Reading Esther's book is like hanging with a supersavvy, whip-smart girlfriend over cocktails—okay, Pinot Noir—as she dishes and dispels dietary myths, and provides an easy-to-implement path to staying lean and sexy for life. Just like a fabulous brunch with my best girlfriends, I didn't want *Cavewomen Don't Get Fat* to end.

Introduction

For most of my life, I've hated the word *diet*. I'm not a fan of the word for many reasons, but mostly because no "diet" has ever worked for me. I've just never figured out how to reconcile eating "diet foods" with living a happy and balanced life.

Does this sound familiar?

Most women I work with feel the same way: when we hear the word *diet*, we quickly duck into a hidden place of shame, where we secretly know we'll fail—despite our best efforts. That's because most diets try to force us into a kind of submission—*Eat this! Avoid that!*—that undermines everything we know to be true about being confident, healthy, independent women.

For me, like many of you, there's nothing worse than putting all of our past failures aside and making a commitment to this or that diet, only to find that, after initially losing weight (and usually suffering in the process), the pounds that we diligently shed (usually due to a degree of willpower that is unsustainable) find their way back to us. Oh, and I'm sure you noticed that those lost-and-gained pounds usually bring a few new pounds home with them.

It's high time we throw up our hands and admit that trying to lose weight the "traditional" way just doesn't work. But what then? Should we just resign ourselves to the fact that we may be carrying around five, ten, twenty, or more pounds that keep us from feeling as sexy and healthy as we deserve to feel? Do we settle for mercurial mood swings, constant food cravings, terrible PMS or scorching hot flashes, foggy brains, and low energy? Or do we toss the notion of dieting out the window and decide that we're just going to simplify our lives and finally get back to eating the way we were always designed to do?

It really is that easy. All we need to do is look to our ancestors for the answers. And no, I'm not talking from the time of your great-great-grandma. I'm talking about going way back. Back to the time before smart phones, cars, electricity—even farming. It all begins and ends for us women, nutritionwise and healthwise, back in Paleolithic times.

I discovered that if I follow a diet similar to the one that my long-ago Paleolithic sisters ate, I can be lean, strong, sexy, and healthy. Forever. And you can be too.

And here's why: most diets fail for a reason that may surprise you. It's not because they're so restrictive, which they are, and that's just never any good—especially for someone like me who believes in balance and freedom of choice rather than deprivation. Most diets fail because they sabotage our metabolism by promoting a way of eating (usually low in calories and protein) that ignores how our bodies work.

On a low-calorie diet, your body notices that it's receiving fewer calories, so it sheds some weight initially. While this is happening, your body's ability to produce, distribute, and balance key hormones (the interplay of hormones is what makes up metabolism) efficiently becomes compromised, and though you may lose a few pounds, (or even more than a few), your system is otherwise sent into distress. When this happens, your health—including your body's ability to regulate weight—is thrown out of whack. Your body says, "Okay, gorgeous, it's just a matter of time before you and I either (1) plateau on that particular diet and stop losing weight or (2) throw in the towel and give in to our debilitating hunger, fatigue, moodiness, sleep deprivation, cravings, and other symptoms of metabolic distress.

It seems that our ancestors didn't suffer from this kind of metabolic trauma. Instead, they ate for fuel and were rewarded with the physical strength, stamina, and body health they needed to make it to the next day.

I've been a holistic nutritionist in New York City for nearly two decades, and, believe me, I've seen every fad diet out there. But the Paleo diet, which has been around for millions of years, works, especially when it's adapted by someone like me, who understands how to tweak these ancient principles and apply them to our modern lives, which are fast, complicated, fun, and, at times, pretty overwhelming.

Paleo meets feminine in my Paleo Chic plan, which is custom tailored to meet the ancient needs of the modern woman. Eating like our human ancestors did is particularly effective for today's modern woman who wants to be slim, toned, and fit. The Paleo diet you've heard so much about isn't just for hard-core CrossFitters and meat-loving men. By eating like a cavewoman, you'll enjoy foods that are protein rich, hormone balancing, detoxifying, and satisfying.

My Paleo Chic diet is the ultramodern version of the Paleo diet that is specifically tailored to the nutritional, hormonal, and real world needs of women like you and me. It is a three-step evolution in achieving transformation.

The Paleo Detox plan, which is the first phase, hits the metabolic reset button by clearing out extra sugar and extra carbs. Doing so will quench your inner inflammatory fires and let your body release extra water and bloat. You'll also give your gut, or intestinal tract, a rest and help it start to repair itself by clearing out allergenic foods that are causing you to pack on extra weight.

The Paleo Reset plan gently reintroduces carbs to sustain your energy and throws you a bone with an optional "cheat meal." You will still continue on your weight loss path in this phase, with the addition of a complex starch in your day.

And the Paleo Chic plan lets you live gorgeously as a modern cavewoman and maintain your physique with a whole-foods, balanced, clean way of eating. Within the Paleo Chic realm, you can enjoy up to two complex starches per day and up to two cheat meals per week for the uber-active exercisers.

Most diets take a one-size-fits-all approach; my plan lets you custom tailor the program to your individual needs. And it will give you the tools to streamline your relationship to food and streamline your body. Think of carbs as your metabolic modulators on this plan: eating less generates faster results; eating more generates slower results. Your energy levels, workouts, and changes in overall body fat will all dictate the role that carbs play in your everyday food choices and in changing your physique. And when you understand the relationship that they have with your body, you can finally get the results you're looking for—for good.

I've watched, gratified and humbled, how the Paleo Chic plan has transformed the lives of hundreds of my clients, start to finish.

Now it's time for you to reap the benefits of the Paleo Chic plan too.

The Paleo Chic diet will help you:

boost your energy;
balance your hormones naturally;
burn fat;
stabilize your brain biochemistry and gain control over
    cravings;
promote digestive health and improve nutrient absorption;
build lean muscle mass;
sleep deeply and restoratively;
manage and reduce stress;
detoxify your body; and
improve your hormonal balance and metabolic functioning.

The Paleo Chic diet is not about:

calorie counting;
low-fat dieting;

living with hunger and cravings;

having to engage in high-impact fitness regimens that are hard
    to sustain;

forfeiting muscle for weight loss;

promoting processed foods; and

abusing your body (or soul) in any way.

Your body knows what it needs to function optimally—in fact, it's known for a very, very long time. And I know that you can heal your body with food. All you need to bring to the table is your willingness to be the best, sexiest, sveltest, and healthiest you possible. If you follow my plan, you'll lose those annoying extra pounds, build lean muscle mass, and feel like the gorgeous goddess you are meant to be.

Here are the benefits that the Paleo Chic diet can help you achieve:

- You can eat plenty of food and lose weight.
- You will not feel hungry or experience overwhelming cravings, because you will eat three healthful meals and two nutritious snacks every day.
- Your body can become the lean, mean fighting machine that it is designed to be.
- You will lose fat and gain lean muscle mass.
- Your skin will glow.
- Your blood sugar levels will remain steady, so you won't crash and burn or have nasty mood swings.
- You will enjoy deep, restorative sleep.
- Your body and mind will be better able to cope with and ward off stress.
- Most importantly, eating like a Paleo cavewoman will ground you in a very deep, authentic way of living that will free up your most valuable and vital resources.

. . .

If you're like me, though, jumping into the deep end with anything radically new can be a recipe for disaster. I've found that when I approach a major lifestyle change patiently, I have a better chance of sustaining that change over the long term and thus setting myself up for success. That's why I encourage any of you who want to lose weight, feel more energetic, balance your hormones, and just be healthier to try my Paleo Chic diet for a month. That's all. Just give it four weeks. I feel confident that by making this minimal commitment to detox your body and eat delicious, clean food, you will want to make this a way of life.

During the first month, I'm going to encourage you to give your body a fighting chance at health by ditching all those toxic processed foods—soda, candy, crackers, snack foods, and so on— that you may have been feeding yourself. I'll also ask you to look at your sleep habits and commit to getting adequate, rejuvenating rest each night. I'll also coach you to de-stress your life as best you can, too. I'll show you how to increase your intake of lean, healthy proteins while reducing your intake of carbohydrates (especially the processed kind). I'll ask you to be extra nice to yourself, because it takes time—and a lot of compassion—to unlearn all of our modern eating habits.

How do I know all of this? Been there, done that. Now that I eat like a cavewoman, I've never felt and looked better.

Before you make any changes at all, take a photograph of yourself just as you are now. Have your body fat measured by a strength coach or nutritionally oriented physician who knows how to use body fat calipers to determine your current muscle-to-fat ratio. When the first thirty days are up, I want you to take another picture and recheck your caliper measurements. I think you'll be stunned by how much you will have already begun to transform yourself.

The Paleo Chic diet will improve your overall health and quality of life. So I hope that you embrace these changes and think of them as giving your body a gift for the rest of your life. As you embark upon creating your own Paleo kitchen, you may need to initially prepare meals that are different from the ones your family typically eats until everyone gets on board. That's all okay, and it's part of this process. I want to encourage you to be as passionate as possible about this way of eating, because I know how well the Paleo Chic plan works. Each and every one of us has unlimited potential to build lean muscle, burn body fat, and stoke our metabolic fire. The changes in your body will come with time, but the first step lies in changing how you *feel*.

Cavewomen Don't Get Fat is about where we're at right now societally. Now more than ever we need to go back to the land and clear our bodies of the fake-food clutter. We need to understand that millions of years of evolution can't be wrong, and that returning to our roots will restore our health, balance hormones, revitalize energy, and burn fat. It's exactly the wake-up call we women need to reclaim our forgotten bodies. Let's get started!

PART 1

Gorgeous Girls Gone Wild

CHAPTER 1

Looking Good Is in Your Genes

I f you're like most women (including me, of course), over your lifetime, you've tried at least three to five different diets—without experiencing lasting success from any of them. The American dieting industry has blossomed into a multibillion-dollar-a-year behemoth that thrives on desperate women who will try anything to lower that number on their scales. Our cultural obsession with "dieting" makes us vulnerable to counting points or calories, having low-calorie meals delivered to our doors, or drinking "cleansing" drinks five times a day. Yet we're still overweight, stressed out, unhealthy, and exhausted.

The plain truth is that our modern lifestyle and the foods that are aggressively marketed to us are making our bodies and us sick, fat, bloated, and unrecognizable. It's time to revisit our foundations as human animals and fuel our bodies in ways that are more in synch with the natural world. Sometimes in order to move forward, we have to be willing to look back. If you've learned this the hard way and have spent most of your life chasing one fad diet after another, I've got your number. But you need a game changer. It's time to stop what you are doing and listen to your body. I have spent years looking at all the medical literature and data that show that

a diet high in lean proteins and low in unhealthy carbohydrates—
yes, there are healthy carbs: vegetables and fruit—will keep us lean,
healthy, and metabolically at our peak.

My Paleo Chic diet offers a three-way mirror that lets you look
at the effect of how you nourish yourself from all angles. You'll look
gorgeous from every angle, too.

Evolution Comes Full Circle

Our species—or, more specifically, the human body—did not
evolve to run on "fuels" such as chips, candy, and prepackaged cakes
and meals. We aren't equipped for highly processed foods that are
loaded with bad fats, sugar, salt, and unpronounceable chemicals. In
fact, our metabolic needs have changed little over the past ten thousand years, and our bodies—reliable systems that they are—still
function best when they're fueled with whole, unprocessed foods.
In other words, Paleolithic people would not have done well on a
diet of McDonald's, either. Instead, our ancestors ate what was fresh
and at hand: whether it was game, fruit, nuts, seeds, vegetables, or
fish. We were hunters and gatherers, not fast-food chasers. Since
there was no refrigeration way back then, our diets were primarily
made up of fresh, nutrient-dense foods that were rich in vitamins,
minerals, fiber, protein, and other crucial fuel generators.

I'm not saying that Paleolithic people were disease-free or
lived longer than we do. (As a point of fact, the lifespan of Paleolithic people was pretty short, due to the "eat or be eaten" nature
of human existence back then.) But we do know that Paleolithic
people ate to live—which is all our bodies really need us to do. If we
can remember this, and if we can strip away all of the temptations
we face from engineered foods in pretty packaging and eat in order
to live as well as we possibly can, we'll approach food as medicine
rather than as comfort, stress relief, drugs, or distractions, and we'll
be oh-so-much better and better-looking for it.

In other words, the simpler the better. That's the core message and principle of the Paleo Chic diet.

The Paleo Chic plan helps you to reboot your metabolism in ways that will do your body and mind more good than you can imagine: losing weight and gaining health. It's all about learning to work with—not against—your body, to listen to its ancient, evolved wisdom. Instead, it's about giving that awesome body of yours exactly what it needs.

The Paleo Chic diet is designed to support and enhance your genetic potential, and the net benefit is an improvement in your overall health and well-being. I know how it rolls. Because I'm often in a cocktail state of mind, I've found that the Paleo Chic plan allows me to "live hard, play hard," and because of it, I feel (and look) better than I ever have.

Let's be clear that I'm not perfect on it, and the truth is, I don't want to be. I know I can go out with my friends for Saturday-night drinks and dinner and wake up the next day and hit the ground running because the Paleo Chic plan has taught me how to strike a balance between the big picture and the moments of decadent fun that we all need. I can let loose from time to time, without any of the guilt and without losing my sense of well-being. It's a pretty gorgeous thing.

PALEO CHIC TERMS

Here's a handy list of Paleo words and terms used throughout the book:

Carbohydrates. A component of foods that supplies energy (calories) to the body and has the greatest influence on your body's ability to burn fat. The three broad categories of carbohydrates are sugars (also called simple carbohydrates), starches (also called complex carbohydrates), and fiber. Except for fiber and resistant starch, which resists digestion and acts like dietary fiber, carbohydrates cause a higher and faster rise in blood glucose (sugar)—the body's chief source of fuel—than proteins and fats do. Berries, apples, pears, spinach, kale, Brussels sprouts, sweet potatoes, winter squash, rutabagas, parsnips, turnips, and jicamas are all carbs that won't tip the fat-burning scales.

Cavewoman. Although the modern woman isn't really a cavewoman, she can certainly eat like one. This means that she can hunt and gather locally grown produce, livestock, poultry, fish, and eggs. It also means she steers clear of processed foods filled with chemicals, artificial colors, flavors, sweeteners, and genetically modified organisms, or GMOs (explained on page 51). A cavewoman uses natural skin care and cleaning products, and lives as natural a life as she can under modern circumstances and the influence of technology and social norms.

Clean Eating. Clean eating is a lifestyle choice. When someone decides to "eat clean" she eliminates all processed foods and additives from her diet. In other words, you are choosing to eat whole, unrefined foods that have not been altered in any way and are as close to their natural state as possible. Nowadays, this means eating foods with five or fewer ingredients—all of which are pronounceable. Eating clean has many benefits, including weight loss, clear skin, improved energy, deep sleep, and a lean body composition.

Clean foods have many definitions in my home. The first is in its preparation. I wash all fruits and vegetables in a 3-to-1 solution of water to vinegar to remove pesticides from conventionally grown produce. I also wash under running water any foods wrapped in plastic, such as meat, poultry, and fish. I have my meats packaged in butcher paper whenever possible, *sans* plastic, and store food in glass containers with snap-on lids. Clean foods are minimally processed, meats are grass fed until they're taken to market, and fruits and vegetables are grown locally and/or organically—in other words, foods that walked, flew, swam, or grew from the ground (or trees).

Fats. Fats are both a major form of energy and a delicious addition to any food. Butter, heavy cream, olive and coconut oils, raw nuts and nut butters, and avocadoes all had me at hello. The right fats can combat PMS, migraines, coronary artery disease, diabetes, and obesity; hydrogenated oils like margarine that contain trans fats and poor-quality oils such as soybean, corn, canola, and cottonseed can make you inflamed, arthritic, obese, and depressed.

Hormones. Hormones are biochemical messengers produced by the endocrine organs that control bodily functions such as growth, sexual development and reproduction, weight control, stress, and sleep. Cortisol, a stress hormone produced by the adrenal glands, can either build or break down muscle. Estrogen and progesterone regulate sexual development, menstrual cycles, and fertility; testosterone helps build lean muscle (yes, women's bodies do make some testosterone); and dehydroepiandrosterone (DHEA) works in conjunction with the reproductive hormones to support fertility. Leptin and ghrelin regulate hunger and fullness. Growth hormone (GH) supports the production of lean muscle mass.

Metabolism. Metabolism encompasses all the chemical processes that occur within the body to keep us functioning. How well we eat, how active we are, and how many toxins we're exposed to determine how well our metabolism runs.

Neocarb. A neocarb is a carbohydrate introduced to the human diet within the last ten thousand years with the advent of modern agriculture. Think grains, legumes, and soy.

Paleocarb. Paleocarbs are carbohydrates that have existed since the beginning of time. They include vegetables, nuts, seeds, and fruits. These carbs are considered healthy because they contain antioxidants and fiber and are relatively low in sugar.

Protein. Proteins make up our cells, skin, hair, nails, and every organ and tissue in our bodies. The dietary protein we eat helps rebuild and repair the proteins in our bodies. Paleo-friendly proteins include pastured meats, poultry, fish, eggs, and wild game. Although our bodies can make some amino acids—organic compounds that are essential to cell growth and maintenance and to all metabolic processes—they also require that we eat protein from outside sources to get the rest.

CHAPTER 2

The Nutritional Benefits of the Paleo Chic Diet

Here's a simple fact: unprocessed foods such as fresh fruits and vegetables, lean meats and fish always—and I mean always—contain fewer calories than processed foods. Think about that for a moment. Actually, stop and think about what, exactly, a calorie is.

A calorie is a unit of energy. It's a way for us to get a sense of the energy value that is contained within each food. You would think, then, that a calorie would be a constant, set unit of measurement—and it is—but, really, it's not. Huh? Bear with me here. A calorie from one food source doesn't always have the nutritional value of a calorie from another, less healthful food source. It's just a fact that some calories are better than others.

Do you think your body processes the 100 calories you find in say, a candy bar, the way it does the 100 calories you get from a salad made with organic produce or the 100 calories in a slice of roasted organic chicken? The answer is a resounding no: what comes along with those calories—those units of energy—has a great impact on how your body actually deals with those calories. That's why there's currently such an outcry about highly processed foods that are marketed as "no fat" or "low fat." These alleged diet foods are filled with sugars, salt, and unhealthy fat substitutes, yet because they're packaged in "low-calorie" *servings*, we're mislead to believe that they're somehow good for our bodies. Oh, if this were only true! But it's not.

One of the great upsides to the Paleo Chic diet is that you will be able to eat plenty of healthy calories and still lose weight. That's because these foods are rich in nutrient-dense calories, as opposed to empty calories. You'll be eating in order to ignite your metabolism, not to tamp it down. Becoming Paleo Chic means that eating well—and abundantly—is a good thing, because your gorgeous body will be fueled as well as satisfied.

In addition to emphasizing nutrient-dense calories, the Paleo Chic diet is designed to support, balance, and enhance the body's incredibly vital metabolic systems. Think of your metabolic system as a network of highly specialized channels of communication. (It's like the Wi-Fi your body runs on.) Give your metabolism the right information—no spam—and the communication comes through clearly and effectively.

Our Bodies are Pretty Effin' Efficient

Since our bodies are governed by our metabolic systems, it makes sense that we would want to fill them with the best fuel possible. To do this, we need to understand what it is our bodies need.

Our bodies, as a rule, are designed to run on fewer carbohydrates than most of us are accustomed to eating. When you reduce the number of carbs you consume, your metabolism runs much more efficiently. You will likely see an immediate improvement in your moods, your energy levels, your sleep patterns, and your mental focus. Eating neocarbs is like putting sludgy, viscous fuel into a system that wants something clear and fluid. Also, neocarbs are highly corrosive to your metabolic components (think of them as causing your system to rust), so those of us who want to be hot and active must avoid these fuels at all costs.

By lowering our carb intake, we encourage our bodies to burn stored sugars (glycogen) and this, in turn, encourages our bodies to let go of fat. When this happens, it's as if our communication channels open wide, and our vital organs can then perform their duties well. Suddenly we find ourselves feeling much, much better.

When you learn to eat the Paleo Chic way, you will find that it becomes nearly impossible to overeat. You will find that you're rarely or ever feeling hungry. Those cravings at ten in the morning or three in the afternoon will disappear. Filling up on healthy carbs (fresh fruits and veggies) will go a long way toward reducing your cravings for highly processed foods. And this is a big part of why the Paleo Chic plan is so healthful. The processed sweets that are aggressively marketed to us are major "trigger" foods that are actually engineered to elicit cravings in us. Mother Nature, thank our stars and garters, isn't a major corporation that puts profits over people, so by eating Paleo Chic, we not only nip those cravings but also get to keep some cold cash in our pockets. And that is a beautiful thing.

Burn, Baby, Burn

Optimal fat loss is a metabolic process by which your body breaks down fat in favor of building lean muscle. When your hormones are balanced, the body naturally engages in regular fat burning, which leads to appetite control and level states of mood and energy. When we eat solely to support our metabolism, we sleep well, awake refreshed, feel energized, and have better mental acuity. Carrying excess fat stymies our metabolic systems. The Paleo Chic diet "restarts" our metabolic circuitry so that our bodies can shed unwanted fat and function more optimally.

The best way to support the body's efforts to burn fat is through clean eating. What and when you eat will determine how well you burn fat, and understanding this basic principle is the foundation to all weight loss. I would even go so far as to say that your diet is responsible for 80 percent of weight loss (with exercise accounting for 20 percent). Every time one of my clients says, "I eat a healthy diet, but I am not losing weight. Why not?" I know that she is eating the wrong kinds of healthy foods. Not all healthy foods prompt the fat-burning command metabolically. When you're not fueling for fat burning and muscle building, it doesn't matter how much you exercise, you won't lose weight.

Here's a cavewoman truth: every bit of food you eat either puts your body in a fat-burning or fat-storing state. It's up to you to decide which one you prefer.

The Skinny on Skinny-Fat

Skinny-fat means that a woman has too much fat (especially belly fat) and not enough muscle, even though the number on her scale indicates that she's in that magical range called "thin." In spite of her numbers looking good on the outside, she's probably suffering from the effects of a sluggish, poorly fueled metabolism on the inside, just like her overweight girlfriends. *Mon Dieu!* you think. How is this possible?

It all depends on the source and type of calories that our "skinny-fat" girl is consuming. If her diet consists of empty calories that are high in sugar and low in protein, she won't be giving her body the building blocks it needs to build lean muscle mass. This girl might look good in clothes, but ask her to sprint, lug a heavy bag, or move a bookshelf, and she won't be able to do it. And guess what else? In spite of a thin physique, she may still be jiggly and even have cellulite. The take-home lesson here is that even if you're "thin," you still need to eat a diet that is high in fat-burning, muscle-building calories. Otherwise you won't achieve the cavewoman fierceness we all need to embrace all that life has to offer.

Other Benefits of Eating Paleo Chic

Aside from shedding any unwanted fat and building lean muscle mass, the Paleo Chic diet reduces systemic inflammation (another form of metabolic corrosion) that can manifest as extra body fat, migraines, PMS, joint aches, and irritable bowel, to name a few examples. It also improves digestion, clears out our sinuses, and improves our cardiovascular health. It offers as much hormonal support to women who are in the throes of the childbearing years as it does to women entering—or beyond—menopause. And this is important, because the "symptoms" we've been led to believe are unavoidable at menopause aren't normal at all: there is no reason why any of us should suffer from hot flashes, weight gain, night sweats, vaginal dryness, or brain fog when our hormones undergo such a natural shift. These symptoms are, I believe, the result of a lifetime of loading our bodies with unhealthy carbs and foods that are not clean. This includes overly processed grains (this is the reason why gluten intolerance is on the rise in this country), too much dairy, and way, way too much sugar. Ditching these toxic "foods" from our diets will reduce not just the symptoms of menopause, but the symptoms of PMS too.

The Paleo Chic diet reduces the phytic acid in our lives. Phytic acids are the indigestible forms of phosphorous found in plants and seeds: along with being impossible to digest, they block the body's ability to absorb other, desirable nutrients that are ingested with them. Making sure that we get an adequate intake of trace minerals (such as zinc, magnesium, calcium, and iron) by cleaning up the gut and reducing phytic acid is essential to maintaining strong bones and building lean muscle. They also help regulate our hormonal fluctuations (and so affect our menstruation cycles) and are crucial for core metabolic regulation.

If nuts are so good for us but contain as much (if not more) phytic acid than beans and grains, why are they allowed on the Paleo Chic plan? There is a case to be made here for a dietary loophole with nuts, because they are typically eaten as a condiment, not as a side or main dish. So if you respect your Paleo ancestors and think about limiting your intake of nuts to an amount equal to what could be found in nature, you're good to go. Small quantities of nuts (¼ cup max) should not throw you too off-kilter. You are also welcome to soak your nuts in a covered bowl of salt water for twelve hours to reduce the levels of phytic acid. After the soak, rinse the nuts in a colander and dry them by placing them in a single layer on a baking sheet or in a dehydrator. Set the temperature to 120°F for twelve hours. Store nuts in an airtight container in the freezer for optimal freshness.

My Paleo Chic diet also flips the bird to "fake" fats like margarine and trans fats and instead encourages eating an appropriate amount of healthy fats (such as those found in grass-fed beef) so that your body can properly produce hormones. The Paleo Chic diet also honors and helps restore the optimal ratio of the fatty acids omega-3 and omega-6 (see page 85), by cutting hydrogenated oils (which are high in O-6) from your diet and instead using oils that promote vivacious health, such as fish oil, which is high in O-3.

Losing Weight the Paleo Way

The key to losing weight boils down to a few very simple, ancient dietary guidelines:

- Eat high-quality lean proteins such as pastured poultry, grass-fed beef, and wild fish.

- Select your fats carefully. For example, olive oil and butter are fine, but no trans fats and no hydrogenated oils.
- Naturally occurring carbohydrates include fiber- and nutrient-dense fruits and vegetables.

These are the very foods that sustained our hunting-and-gathering ancestors who ate what they could catch, pluck, or dig up. We need to step away from neocarbs, which are the overengineered results of our agricultural "progress" (enriched flour products, sugar-infused drinks and foods, genetically beefed-up grains and animal products). We need to step away from factory-generated food and move, instead, back into the bush.

Why is this so imperative? Because eating sixty pounds of grain and thirty pounds of sugar—as the typical American does each year—is making us fat, sick, and tired. We're overindulging on highly processed foods to the tune of about four and a half pounds per week. It seems pretty clear to me that the "modern" approach, at least where dietary health is concerned, has got it all wrong.

By eating lean protein, the most important macronutrient, you will support your body's chemistry in the best way possible. Protein provides slow, steady energy, helps you feel full, and keeps blood sugar levels calm—ditto your mood and your hormones. Think of protein as the calming base nutrient that supplies what your cells need most to thrive. Organic, fresh, and local sources of protein also support bone and skin. (Our bodies love both calcium and collagen.)

Protein packs a wallop, so we don't need to overindulge on the Paleo Chic diet: instead, we like to enjoy our protein with an array of colorful, local, organic produce that rounds out our nutritional needs by infusing our bodies with nutrients, vitamins, minerals, fibers, and the kinds of sugars and carbs we actually need.

On this plan, I encourage you to ditch those high-gluten foods (all types of grains, including foods made with wheat, rye, oats, spelt, and others) that are known to cause allergies, inflammation, and weight gain, and instead focus on vegetables and fruits. Color is key, and the more natural color you bring to the plate, the healthier your diet will be.

When you become a modern-day cavewoman, you protect yourself from the toxins that are found in all types of processed foods, including pesticides, chemicals, dyes, preservatives, hormones, and other artificial ingredients. Your body will be able to focus on breaking down the healthful components of the whole foods you'll be taking in, rather than scrambling to ward off the ill effects caused by the myriad harmful ingredients that are hidden in processed foods.

CHAPTER 3

Don't Let Stress Weigh You Down

I recently saw a graphic that perfectly illustrates the metabolic differences between men and women. On one side of the page there is a light switch and the caption under it says "Man." On the other side of the page is an image of a complex circuit board, of the kind you might find, say, inside the computer that runs the Space Shuttle. Under this image is the word "Woman."

The female metabolic systems—more specifically, our hormones—are very much like that circuit board: sophisticated, very complex, and quite delicate. When it comes to our bodies, our hormones (as we all know) can either work for us or against us. Once any number of them—or even one, for that matter—gets out of whack, there's a domino effect, and before you know it, you just feel like crap. Left unchecked, any kind of hormonal imbalance makes losing weight, getting enough sleep, or functioning well in our jobs or our lives impossible. I would go so far as to argue that managing our hormones is the number one preventative health measure any of us can take. Your holistic physician can test these for you and suggest making healthy lifestyle changes accordingly.

I'm going to outline the three basic groups of hormones we need to be aware of:

1. insulin and cortisol: the fat-burning superstar hormones;
2. the mighty thyroid and adrenal hormones; and
3. estrogen and progesterone: the female hormones that dictate the cycles of our lives.

I've prioritized these hormones in this order, because I've found that by addressing numbers 1 and 2, number 3 rebalances as a result.

First, let's make sure we're all clear on what, exactly, hormones are. In a nutshell, they're the biochemical messengers produced in our glands that control all sorts of bodily processes, including prompting cell and bone growth, raising and lowering blood sugar levels, dictating sexual development, making reproduction possible, cuing fat burning and muscle development, regulating sleep, and orchestrating stress management. Not to mention making sure our brains function well. Understanding hormone production and balance is essential to the Paleo woman who wants to look and feel her best—at any age.

1. Insulin and Cortisol: The Fat-Burning Superstar Hormones

While estrogen and progesterone are the key female hormonal players, two other hormones are critical when it comes to losing weight and feeling great. The first is insulin, produced by the pancreas, which regulates blood sugar. Adequate insulin production is essential for metabolizing carbohydrates and fat, and telling the body's cells to absorb glucose from the circulation for energy. The second is cortisol, often referred to as the stress hormone because it is overproduced when our bodies are under too much stress. Cortisol is like insulin, crucial to metabolizing fat, protein, and calcium.

In order to keep these two key hormones in balance, there are two basic principles that all cavewomen must follow: eat fewer starchy carbohydrates (in this book, simple carbs equal sugar) and minimize stress in your life. Only when you address these two big issues will your body be able to give up unwanted fat. I know, easier said than done, but that's what becoming a cavewoman is all about.

Insulin works to eliminate or store fat, depending on how much sugar needs to be moved through your system. Too much sugar in your bloodstream will be converted into fat. If you eat less sugar, the insulin your pancreas produces helps produce lean muscle rather than having to manage all that sugar; think of it as the anabolic, or muscle-building, holy grail. When you eat too much sugar, you cue your body to produce too much insulin. When you've got too much insulin coursing through your circulation you will gain weight and decrease your body's ability to burn fat.

The beauty of taking charge of your insulin levels is this: if your pancreas is able to produce insulin efficiently, you can control your insulin levels by diet alone. Those with type 2 diabetes (noninsulin-dependent) know that the frontline medical treatment is diet and that, often, with the right kind of dietary modifications, they can forego having to take medications to manage the disease.

Cortisol production also responds well to lifestyle changes, and this is where exercise and rest come into play. When we engage in physical activity—walk, run, lift weights—we elevate our cortisol levels for the right reasons as opposed to those brought on by external forms of stress. We exercise, produce just the right amounts of cortisol, then rest, and bring down those levels. This kind of healthful cycling of cortisol promotes the development of lean muscle, which is essential to losing fat.

On the flip side, if we're chronically under the gun (with work and responsibilities at home or a combination of these) we overproduce cortisol, which sends our body into a kind of shock that yells "Hey, everyone, pump your brakes!" This means that our bodies then grasp onto the fat that we're trying to shed, almost like a parent holding on to a cocktail for dear life after a long day with screaming kids.

When our systems are drenched in cortisol, we can't think straight, we don't sleep well, our eating deteriorates, and we get—or stay—fat.

2. The Mighty Thyroid and Adrenal Hormones

The next biggest movers of female physiology are thyroid, adrenaline, and noradrenaline hormones. They're essential for producing estrogen and progesterone.

The thyroid makes and releases two hormones: triiodothyronine (T_3) and thyroxine (T_4). The thyroid's main job is to produce the right amount of thyroid hormone to regulate metabolism, heart rate, body temperature, digestion, and muscle strength. The adrenal glands make the hormones adrenaline and noradrenaline (epinephrine) that allow you to respond to all kinds of stress. Both the thyroid and the adrenal glands act in conjunction with each other as guardians of the endocrine system. They are constantly responding to ever-changing conditions within the body due to their complex set of sensors. Under stress, the brain tells the adrenal glands to make cortisol, which will inhibit the conversion of T_4 to T_3. If you've been under stress for years, you can be more prone to hypothyroidism (underactive thyroid). Balancing your stress, eating lots of quality proteins, sleeping from ten o'clock until six, and popping some supplements can help your body hit the reset button on your metabolism. Refer to the "Cortisol Control" protocol in chapter 11 for more information.

If your insulin and cortisol levels are high, and your thyroid and adrenal glands are dysfunctional, changing your estrogen and progesterone levels won't make a dent in getting you lean. The minute you start addressing insulin and cortisol and the adrenal-thyroid axis, the estrogen and progesterone levels will take care of themselves. If you try to change your biochemistry by starting with estrogen and progesterone management first, your efforts will be wasted. And if you don't control your stress, you're also going to be hard pressed to get your thyroid functioning up to speed. But, if you can reduce your stress, you'll elevate your thyroid function. And that is where the magic happens.

3. Estrogen and Progesterone: The Female Hormones That Dictate the Cycles of Our Lives

Estrogen is actually the name of a class of hormones. The three major estrogens produced by women are estriol, estradiol, and estrone. Estrogens are steroid hormones that are responsible for sexual development in girls, an increase in body fat during development, and helping to keep bones strong. This delicate hormonal ecosystem helps a girl's body prepare for menstrual cycles and carry children down the road.

Progesterone is also a steroid hormone. The ovaries produce the majority of progesterone, but only when ovulation occurs. As we approach menopause, our progesterone wanes. This deficiency is responsible for many of the symptoms associated with menopause, such as sleep disruption, weight gain, foggy thinking, and joint and bone inflammation. When our progesterone levels drop, our bodies become estrogen dominant. The Paleo Chic diet helps correct this imbalance.

How to Stay in Balance

To understand how we women produce and store fat, you need to know what happens hormonally during our monthly cycle. During the first fourteen days, estrogen levels peak and then fall. Progesterone lies low for this first half of the cycle, and then spikes up and crashes back down during the second half. So the first half of the cycle is estrogen heavy, while the second half is progesterone rich. Knowing this and eating to keep estrogen and progesterone in balance will help you make healthy food choices that will keep your weight and the rest of your metabolism on an even keel. Here's how:

- During the first fourteen days of your cycle, known as the follicular phase, you can increase your carbohydrate intake ever so slightly, as long as you also up your cardiovascular activity. Why? Estrogen increases insulin efficacy, and so your body processes sugar more efficiently and is predisposed to retain muscle mass. This means that you're likely to burn, rather than store, fat during this two-week part of your cycle. And that's just what you want to do! Don't go crazy, but it's okay to fan that estrogen fire by increasing your healthy carbohydrate intake slightly. (Think an extra half of a sweet potato here.)
- During the second part of your cycle, the luteal phase, things get a little trickier. As your estrogen levels drop off, your insulin efficiency decreases. Now it's time to cut back on those carbs and cardio, while increasing the amount of protein you eat and do some strength training to reinforce the muscle building that the first half of the month brought.

Women who adjust their diets around the hormonal phases of their cycle report fewer PMS symptoms and less bloating. I personally find that doubling up on protein during the premenstrual phase kicks my cravings to the curb and boosts my energy and mental clarity.

Once you get your period, estrogen and progesterone levels both drop steeply. This is a time when you can be prone to all kinds of crazy cravings, as the drop in our female sex hormones can trigger the neurotransmitters dopamine, serotonin, and gamma-aminobutyric acid (GABA), to misbehave. Stay the course, my Paleo Chic sisters, and you will ride through all of this with ease.

As mentioned above, I find that upping my protein intake at the start of my cycle helps me stay in balance for the entire month.

Adding 2 to 4 ounces of lean meat or fish, an extra egg, or an additional 2 tablespoons of nuts and seeds to each meal will nip those gnarly PMS symptoms in the bud. Increasing your protein consumption will also curb your cravings for carbohydrates and sugars. Protein subdues the hunger center in the hypothalamus—the area of your brain that communicates with your digestive system—while also steadying your blood sugar level.

I'm a believer that chocolate can cure anything, especially the PMS blues. The compounds found in cacao (I'm talking about organic, unsweetened cocoa powder, ladies, not a candy bar) contain phenylethylamine, a substance that controls moods. Phenylethylamine (PEA) mimics the neurotransmitter dopamine and imparts a feeling of well-being and peacefulness. It also contains serotonin, the neurotransmitter that is known to be crucial in keeping depression at bay. So if you get those chocolate cravings at the onset of your cycle, put a heaping tablespoon of organic, unsweetened cocoa powder into a cup of hot water and enjoy.

Upping your physical activity is always a good idea (and very Paleo Chic), but especially when your cycle starts. Exercise tamps down your body's sense that it is under stress, allowing cortisol production to take a breather. Getting any kind of physical activity during this time, be it a leisurely walk, a swim, or a rousing game of tennis, will not only prime your muscles and trip your fat-burning wires, it will clear your head, help you rest, and calm down your hormones.

When the Cycling Stops: Managing Menopause

At some point, we will all hit that time of life when we no longer ride the hormonal roller coaster of the monthly menstrual cycle. However, menopause brings its own hormonal challenges. Once we stop ovulating, progesterone production drops dramatically. At first, we're still producing estrogen, and so this imbalance manifests with a host of symptoms that, on the face of it, look a lot like the symptoms of PMS, but they're not.

Moving into this stage, which tends to be estrogen dominant, we experience hot flashes and night sweats. As our estrogen levels continue to fall, our resistance to insulin increases as our cortisol levels creep up too. This is enough to make any girl cry! You've been thin and glamorous all of your adult life, you do your cardio at the gym, you watch your calories, and all of a sudden your good behavior and habits no longer work for you. Why the change? Because you've always had estrogen and progesterone in your corner diligently working on your behalf. Now, as you become more insulin resistant and more prone to the effects of stress, you find yourself gaining weight. What's a menopausal mama to do? Become a Paleo Chic glamour girl. That's what you do.

If you're postmenopausal and have been eating Paleo but aren't seeing results, you need to work harder to lower your insulin levels. If your current diet includes foods such as sweet potatoes and a lot of fruit and you're not losing weight, it means those foods are no longer working for you. Even healthy starches can prompt insulin overproduction in our bodies, and too much insulin without adequate estrogen is a recipe for fat storage. This is why a high-protein, low-carb Paleo diet will help reset your hormones and get you lean.

"If I go on a low-carb diet, won't I lose muscle?" Although insulin is a fat-storing hormone, it also builds muscle. So if you increase your dietary protein and incorporate a bit of weight training (more on this later) into your regimen three to four times per week, you will not only sustain muscle mass but build it too.

How Stress Disrupts Our Hormones

There is nothing more harmful to healthy hormone production and function than stress. And most of us are under so much stress from one thing or another that we're not even aware of how stressed out we are.

The presence of stress in our lives causes our hormones to push us into a "hyperalert" state, and our systems become flooded with all kinds of mixed messages. The net result is that our endocrine system goes into overdrive, and while it starts pumping out certain hormones to combat stress, other hormones become diluted and depleted. The net effect is that we feel crazy and out of whack, which manifests as anything from uncontrolled PMS, to debilitating symptoms of menopause, such as lethargy and brain fog. When one hormone is overproducing, others literally get drowned out and can't do their jobs. When this happens, our whole system suffers.

Paleo Chic women want no part of this system overload. We're not interested in "having it all" if it means we have to get fat, have lousy skin, lose our sex drive, and feel crazy and depressed in order to do so. The Paleo Chic woman knows that to look and feel good, she has to put her stress-busting cavewoman moves to work.

Tried-and-True Tension Tamers

While clean eating will support your brain biochemistry and fight mood swings and depression, these other lifestyle changes below will take care of the rest. Try one new tension tamer each week to combat stress, which is critical to your overall health. You can also incorporate relaxing activities such as restorative yoga, tai chi, and leisure walking, all of which lower cortisol. While these activities won't burn a lot of calories, the benefits of lowering cortisol will help keep your entire system balanced and set you up to shed fat more easily and effectively.

- Put yourself in a time-out. I'll never forget the time my mother had had enough of my two brothers and me. She looked us all square in the eye, told us she was leaving, got in her car, and drove away. Thankfully, she came back, and when she did, the message was clear: she had been mad as hell, and she wasn't going to take it anymore! Women are wired to overprovide for others; that's just how we roll. But it doesn't mean that we can't take time for ourselves and recharge our batteries. Send the message to your family or those around you and slap a tiara on your head to signal that this is *your* time to check out and to leave you be for the next twenty minutes.
- Boost your oxytocin. Spending time with friends floods your body with oxytocin, a powerful brain modulator that helps you feel happy and calms you down. Oxytocin is also released during breast-feeding and orgasms and helps you mellow out. A girls' night out with your BFFs is a great way to let loose and bond with your fellow cavewomen.
- Take a bath. Light some candles and dump two cups of Epsom salts and ten drops of lavender oil into your bath water. Climb in and read a trashy magazine. Loll, doll! Soak your stress away and take some deep breaths.
- Have a vitamin cocktail daily. The following protocol will help lower your cortisol, promote restful sleep, and keep your energy grooving throughout the day (as a reminder, always consult your nutritionally oriented health care provider before introducing supplements to your diet):

  Omega-3: take two teaspoons (this should be equivalent to 2,000 milligrams [mg]) once a day with food, preferably before you work out.

  Rhodiola rosea: take 200 mg twice a day with food.

  Phosphatidylserine: take 400 mg at bedtime to promote restful sleep.

  Vitamin C: take 2,000 mg immediately following a workout to normalize cortisol.

Chaste tree: take 1,000 mg twice a day of 6:1 extract
to balance the endocrine system and support normal
progesterone levels. Chaste tree can also restore
normal menstrual cycles, especially if you are
amenorrheic and have stopped menstruating.

- Eat wild fish. Wild Alaskan salmon is my favorite. A 6-ounce
serving has almost 700 IU (international units) of vitamin
D and about 2 teaspoons fish oil per serving. The fats
found in omega-3s boost and sustain serotonin levels in
the brain and reduce the vascular inflammation associated
with heart disease. Plus, wild Alaskan salmon contains the
powerful antioxidant astaxanthin, which contains a natural
sun protection factor (SPF) of 5, and the neurotransmitter
DMAE (dimethylaminoethanol), which helps maintain the
gorgeous contours of your face and muscles. Aim to eat
cold-water fatty fish such as salmon, herring, mackerel,
Chilean sea bass, trout, and anchovies at least three times
per week.

- Vitamin O. Let's talk about sex. If you have a secret lover
undercover and are out there having fun, then you know
the joys of spontaneity. A little afternoon delight or sex
on the fly can be quick and dirty and just plain fun! If
you are married or in a long-term relationship, there are
benefits, too: statistics show that married people have
more sex than single people do. But what kind of sex are
we talking about here? Is it mercy sex? Two-pump-chump
sex? A-quickie–before-the-kids-wake-up sex? I'm all for
a quickie, but we need to do better for ourselves. Long,
luscious orgasms have been shown to decrease cortisol
levels and raise the good estrogen (estradiol), and make
your thyroid more efficient. You've got to use it or lose
it. I always tell my husband that it's TV or me. Television
can wait, and that's what the DVR is there for. Break
up your routine and schedule sex around nine at night,

before you and yours are exhausted and too tired to get it up. Or even better, get into bed before you go out on a date—that way, if you stuff your face at dinner, you don't have to worry about getting aroused with a bloated belly afterward!

- Ditch the booze. Grain-based alcohol, beer in particular, increases estrogen and progesterone and decreases testosterone in both men and women. As little as one glass per day can upset your hormonal balance and overall metabolism. If you can't live without your booze each night, have a 4-ounce serving of Pinot or Merlot or a Spanish wine. These wines are rich in resveratrol, which has been shown to inhibit the aromatase enzyme that turns testosterone into estrogen, ultimately lowering estrogen levels.

- Give thanks. I practice gratitude daily and try to instill it in my family members as well. In fact, the mantra in our house has become "A little less attitude, a little more gratitude." Keep a log next to your bed and before you hit the pillow, take two minutes to record three things you were grateful for in your day. Or project gratitude for the beautiful night's sleep you're about to enjoy. Appreciating the beauty of even an ordinary day can naturally lower your anxiety and cortisol levels and end the day on a positive and peaceful note. It will also help you become a happier and kinder person. Remembering just how good we have it can help us keep a healthy perspective on what's important versus what I like to call "high-class problems." Focusing on our blessings frees us up from worry about less important things.

Sleep

According to the American Sleep Institute, 60 percent of Americans say they don't get enough sleep each night. Well, no wonder! We live in a 24/7 society, with our iPads and smart phones on our nightstands. We can shop, be entertained, work, or communicate every minute of every day. A television and a brightly lit clock in the bedroom shut off the body's ability to produce the hormone melatonin, which controls circadian rhythms at night.

Most adults are familiar with the consequences of sleep deprivation: irritability, a case of the three o'clock in the afternoon yawns, lack of mental focus, and—what was I saying? But there's another consequence of sleep deprivation: it can make you fat.

Statistics show that back in the 1960s, the average American slept eight and a half hours per night. Today we sleep fewer than seven hours per night. The rise in obesity has increased significantly during that same period, and the numbers are much more than a coincidence. While toxins play a large role in causing obesity, not getting enough sleep does as well. The less we sleep, the more we weigh.

We know that getting enough sleep builds muscles, facilitates fat burning, reduces cravings and hunger, and gives us better appetite control. Sleep has an even greater impact as a metabolic modulator than food or exercise does, and therefore governs your hormones and your body's ability to lean out. A lack of sleep burns muscle, packs on body fat, and makes us insulin resistant, with the blood work of someone who is obese or diabetic. After just four nights of sleep deprivation, it takes three times more insulin to cause a normal response to carbohydrates in the bloodstream.

We are born with circadian rhythms that dictate our sleep-wake cycles. Circadian rhythms encompass a twenty-four-hour metabolic cycle that is programmed into our genes. These programs are designed to be as metabolically efficient as possible. But what happens when our metabolism is affected by external stimuli and no longer in line with our genetic programming? Our metabolic processes become far less efficient.

We are genetically programmed to work best in daylight. In the daytime, the metabolic processes that control energy, stress, and appetite work best. But after nightfall, these processes become far less efficient. Our appetite gets turned on, so we eat more; our food does not get converted to energy; our stress levels stay elevated; and we gain weight. But when we catch enough z's, we keep our metabolism efficiently running so that we have more energy and actually eat less.

Why You Should Get Plenty of Sleep

Here are four bet-you-didn't-know ways that sleep can help you lose weight.

1. Sleep Makes You Less Hungry. Sleep is critical in controlling fat storage because of the role it plays in regulating hormones. Two hormones in particular rule the roost with appetite regulation: ghrelin and leptin. They're the boss ladies of appetite regulation. Ghrelin says, "I'm hungry," and leptin says, "I've had enough." Ghrelin, secreted in the lining of the stomach, increases hunger; its levels are highest before a meal and lowest after we've eaten. The ideal scenario is the perfect balance between ghrelin and leptin—all achievable on the Paleo Chic plan. Yup, that's right, eating plenty of lean protein suppresses ghrelin and shuts off the hunger mechanism in the brain. And sleep deprivation increases ghrelin and decreases leptin, so a good night's sleep is imperative when fighting the battle of the bulge.

Restricting sleep changes how the brain functions and can cause you to crave that chocolate chip cookie you would otherwise do without. The next time you have a craving, ask yourself how you slept last night!

2. Sleep Decreases Daytime Stress Levels. As you know now, the stress hormone cortisol is a guilty party in contributing to obesity. When our cortisol levels are high, we tend to pack on more fat at the expense of muscle tissue. Sleep plays a major role in cortisol production and our circadian rhythms. Cortisol levels are highest in the morning, to help us get up and out of bed. Once we have breakfast after an overnight fast, the levels fall rapidly. (This is why you must eat breakfast every morning.) Skipping breakfast will raise your cortisol level and keep it elevated for hours, helping you pack on more body fat.

3. Sleep Increases the Body's Ability to Burn Calories. Even if you're following a calorie-restricted diet, you won't make a dent in fat loss until you visit the sandman, because your body will burn fewer calories and pack on more fat no matter how much you limit your food intake. Your appetite will also spiral out of control, and as a result, you'll eat more than your body needs. Worse yet, insomnia is also a cause of insulin resistance, which helps store your food as fat. (See reasons 1 and 2, above.)

Eating lean protein and nuts controls the "I'm hungry" hormone ghrelin, whereas eating sugary snacks spikes it. Control your hunger and cravings with protein and fats and try to head to bed by ten o'clock to reset your hormones.

4. Sleep Increases Muscle Mass. Sleep loss interferes with the body's ability to build muscle mass. Sleep is an anabolic agent because it causes the pituitary gland in the brain to release growth hormone during intervals throughout the night, which stimulates growth and regeneration and supports the production of lean muscle mass. Growth hormone levels are highest when we are young and growing; as we age, the levels drop naturally, and we produce much less (though women do produce more than men). Some people try to delay the effects of aging by injecting themselves with growth hormone, but eating clean foods, sprinting, and strength-building exercises are the best things you can do to produce the juice naturally.

So if you're not producing enough growth hormone because you're not getting enough sleep, you'll lose muscle mass and burn fewer calories and fat throughout the day. In a study with subjects who had been sleep deprived while on reduced-calorie diets, one group slept five and a half hours per night; the other slept eight and a half hours per night. Both groups lost similar amounts of weight, but the group that got a good night's rest lost 50 percent more fat than the sleep-deprived group.

If you want to reclaim your body and set yourself up for success, you'll need to aim for at least seven and a half hours of sleep every night. This may require some lifestyle changes, but if you're serious about slimming down, you need to make the connection between quality sleep and body fat percentages. The number of hours you sleep each night should be consistent throughout the week. Don't bother trying to make up for lost sleep on the weekends; that just isn't enough time to reset your hormones.

How to Get a Good Night's Sleep

- Sit down to breakfast within an hour of waking up and then eat at regular intervals throughout the day, since skipping meals elevates cortisol that can interfere with your nightly sleep.
- Start shutting down for the night (washing your face, brushing your teeth) by nine o'clock to facilitate the release of restorative hormones and insure a good night's sleep.
- If you suffer from anxiety and insomnia at night, do ten minutes of deep-breathing exercises before bed. Lie on your back in bed, place your hands on your stomach, and focus on your breath until you feel your stomach rise and fall under your hands. Breathe in and out through your nose, and count to four with each inhalation and exhalation. Let go of all other thoughts and keep coming back to your breath.

- Avoid stimulants such as ephedra and caffeine. Some people need as much as twenty-four hours to clear 1 cup of morning caffeine from their systems. No caffeine should pass your lips after two in the afternoon if you have trouble sleeping!
- Limit workouts to sixty minutes (unless you are walking, which will lower your cortisol), and try to finish your workout at least four hours before bed. With strength and interval workouts, at the sixty-minute mark, your testosterone levels start to decline and cortisol levels rise—not a good combo for sleeping.
- Meditate. The best part about having a brain is that you can retrain it and create positive changes within yourself. Meditation is one of my favorite ways to rewire, because it promotes a sense of calm and relaxation all day long—even if you do it the night before. The amygdala, an almond-shaped mass of nerve cells deep within the brain, regulates our emotions and is the greatest beneficiary of meditation. If you're feeling anxious, struggling with insomnia, or just craving some deeply restorative and relaxing sleep, practice some guided imagery and form scenarios in your head about places that relax you and watch the magic unfold after a few short days.
- Have an orgasm, either with your partner or by yourself. This will release tension and prompt the flow of feel-good hormones that calm the brain and nourish the nervous system.

Each day presents a new opportunity for us to strive for a good night's sleep. You'll be amazed how your body composition changes once you pair sleep with good nutrition and smart exercise.

PART 2

Modern Myths and Paleo Makeovers

CHAPTER 4

Do These Toxins Make Me Look Fat?

W e've all heard the expression "The road to hell is paved with good intentions." This couldn't be truer than when it comes to trying to lose weight. For many of us, no matter how much we improve our diets or add more exercise classes to our schedules, those three digits on our scales won't budge.

Along with those good intentions, the road to dieting is also paved with harmful toxins that seep into every aspect of our lives. Those toxins are found in the food we eat, the clothes we wear, the technology we use. You name it; toxins are everywhere. We can't see them, we usually can't smell them, and we don't taste them. But they are everywhere, and they undermine our ability to lose weight more than anything else. Because we women carry more body fat than men do, we make better storehouses for toxins. Fat is where they like to hang out. And the more toxic we are, the more fat we store in an effort to dilute those toxins.

Scientists already know that pollutants such as pesticides, fertilizers, and the chemicals found in cleaning products are rapidly moved from the bloodstream and into the body's stored fat. Think of your fat cells as your body's toxic waste dump, the landfill where it tries to hide these chemicals. The more toxins you are exposed to, the harder the body has to work to shuttle these harmful substances away from your vital organs, and the more fat it believes it needs to produce to shield itself from them.

Unfortunately, there is a huge metabolic cost to this kind of toxic garbage hauling and storage: our bodies have to work extremely hard to function under this particularly modern strain. (Cavewomen had all sorts of hazards to worry about, but toxic chemicals wasn't one of them.)

Left to her own devices, Mother Nature does all right by us women. But when we dump toxins into the environment, smoke cigarettes, and use cosmetics, personal care products, and chemical household cleaners, she's going to bite us back. When our bodies hold on to toxins, we become ill in many ways. One example is that our bodies work hard to maintain those fat cells, and this creates a catch-22 situation: our fat-burning mechanisms become sluggish, our appetites increase, and, despite our best efforts to diet, we begin to put on more weight. It's hard to get rid of something (in this case toxin-laced fat) when your body wants to hold on to it so badly. The body refuses to use these fat stores as fuel because that would release the toxins into the circulation, which would be a very bad thing. So although your body may be in survival mode and ultimately trying to protect you, you're not going to like what you see.

But there is a way to rid our bodies of harmful toxins, and we've all heard the term: detoxification. There are very concrete steps we can take to reduce the amount of environmental toxins we are exposed to and to decrease the amount of toxins we ingest with our food.

But before I get into the whys and hows of detoxing, let's chat about how harmful toxins impact the body's ability to lose weight. Our understanding of just how dangerous these substances are has accelerated dramatically in just the past few years. Top-notch scientists and nutritionists have gathered data showing that poor diet and lack of exercise are not the only causes of our obesity epidemic.

There's a rapidly growing body of evidence that links the chemicals found in everything from pesticides, cosmetics, packaging materials (for food and other items), and certain foods to increased fat production. A special word has even been coined by biologist Bruce Blumberg of the University of California at Irvine for these obesity-promoting toxins: obesogens.

You heard right, ladies: there are chemicals strewn all over the environment that are making us fat.

It's believed that obesogens mess with our metabolisms in ways that make our bodies favor fat production and become less efficient at breaking down fats. This is what makes losing weight so difficult for many of us. Interestingly, this toxic trigger for obesity is a particularly American one, given how chemically dependent our society has become since World War II. In many other parts of the world, people eat far less highly processed foods than we do and tend to eat locally grown and raised foods more than we do, too.

Since there's no scientific remedy for restoring your toxin-hijacked metabolism, the best medicine is prevention. And this is where detoxing your environment—and diet—comes into play.

Teasing Out the Toxins That Lurk in Our Kitchens and Homes

You've likely heard the advertising phrase "Better living through chemistry!" Well, if you want to live a long, disease-free life, you need to keep bad chemicals out of your home and your food. Here are some surprising places where toxins are hiding: in the surfaces that make your nonstick pans slick; in the plastic bags, films, wraps, and containers that clog up your kitchen drawers and shelves; and in the water that flows through your kitchen tap. Toxins are also hiding in the food you're lugging home from the grocery store. (High-fructose corn syrup, my gorgeous friends, is a leading obesogen.) They can also be found in the bathroom, beauty, and hair-care products that you use daily. They're even in your plastic shower curtain! So much for washing away the grime of the world: you're actually ingesting it through your scalp and pores pretty much every time you use a brand-name product.

Obesogens are lurking around your yard too: they're in the pesticides and weed killers that keep your grass green and turn your tomatoes red. Unless you're eating all organic foods, they're also showing up on the fruits and veggies you buy at the local grocery store.

And don't get me started on electronic devices. We worry about what those electronic emissions may do to us, but we already know that the heavy metals and plastics that our phones, TVs, and computers are made of are constantly giving off toxic gases.

Feeling overwhelmed? I know—sometimes you have to be scared straight before you take things seriously. I know I do. It's a particularly cavewomanish type of tough love, but you can handle it.

There are obesogens in the medications we take, and in the medications that are fed to the conventionally farmed animals that eventually make it to our dining tables. These compounds make us fat, ruin our libidos, addle our brains (causing headaches, depression, sleep problems), and generally wreak havoc on our endocrine systems. None of this is good for us.

Let's face it: we're not going to give up all of our modern conveniences, but there are some easy things you can do to reduce the obesogen load in your home:

- Get rid of your nonstick cookware; instead, use cast iron, glass, and any other chemically inert cookware, such as clay, stainless steel, and copper pots.
- Toss out the plastic food containers you have and use glass ones instead. Do the same with water bottles, opting for aluminum and glass.
- Minimize eating canned goods. There's a thin layer of toxic plastic inside most cans. Fresh or frozen foods are always

better than canned in terms of lowering your exposure to obesogens.

- When you buy meats, poultry, or seafood, ask that it be wrapped in paper rather than plastic. If you do buy prepackaged foods, rinse them well to wash off any plastic residue before cooking.
- Use a water filter to reduce contaminants in your tap water for drinking. A reverse-osmosis filter is best, but pitchers with carbon filters work well too.
- Try to avoid using aerosols, especially room fresheners and hair sprays. Instead, use organic hair-care products and 100 percent beeswax candles with cotton wicks.
- Use mineral-based cosmetics and organic skin-care products. Ditto shampoos and soaps.
- Use "green" cleaning products and laundry soaps. (See page 267 for a comprehensive list of safe skin-care products and page 269 for a list of household products to use.)
- Give chemicals the finger and switch to organic products free of all forms of BPA (bisphenol A), parfum, propylene glycol, methacrylate, benzaldehyde, octinoxate, isopropyl myristate, polymethyl methacrylate, phthalates, EDTA (ethylenediaminetetraacetic acid), all parabens, any product with sodium lauryl sulfate, butylated hydroxytoluene (BHT), propylene glycol, carbomers, and cocamides.
- Get hot and sweaty in a sauna at least three times per week to facilitate the body's release of toxins. Exercise is another beneficial way to sweat and move out those toxins.

By implementing even just a few of these suggestions, you will begin to detoxify, and you will give your body a fighting chance to shed some weight. For a more comprehensive lifestyle guide to toxins, treat yourself to Debra Lynn Dadd's amazing book *Home Safe Home: Protecting Yourself and Your Family from Everyday Toxics and Harmful Household Products.*

Food as Medicine: Detoxifying Your Diet

Now that you've started to kick environmental toxins to the curb, it's time to get the dirty stuff out of your diet too.

When we work consciously to avoid ingesting toxins, we prime our bodies to lose weight, lower our risks of getting hormone-related illness (such as diabetes, certain cancers, heart disease), and improve our moods, our sex drive, and, of course, our overall energy.

What we put into our bodies matters. We know that some items are no-nos because they make us fat and, even worse, sick. Every Paleo Chic woman banishes tobacco, eliminates refined sugars, and cuts way, way back on her alcohol consumption. (Of course, indulging in a celebratory cosmopolitan or margarita now and then is fine.) We also go easy on caffeine and strive to buy organic, fresh, grass-fed, and local foods whenever possible.

Here are other Paleo Chic ways to protect yourself from toxic overload:

- Eat your greens. Dark leafy greens and bright green vegetables are like free-radical-seeking drones: they're rich in chlorophyll and help keep our livers functioning at their highest capacity.
- Pile your plate with fresh fruits, vegetables, and herbs in a rainbow of colors. Color indicates the presence of vitamins and minerals, and the more vibrant they are, the more toxin-fighting power they have.
- Eat organic. Believe it or not, it takes only a week of eating all-organic to allow your body to eliminate the pesticide residue that it may have built up. Even if you can't buy organic all the time, doing so as much as possible will do your body a world of good.
- Up your antioxidant intake by eating more berries, cruciferous vegetables (broccoli, cauliflower, bok choy,

watercress, cabbage), dark green vegetables, tomatoes, avocados, and nuts. Think of antioxidants as nature's firemen. They'll tap out inflammation, which can manifest as joint pain and skin conditions such as psoriasis and acne. They promote cell growth and help create a cellular barrier to free radicals, which are like little pinballs that seek electrons from other cells in order to make themselves more stable. These free radicals accelerate aging, initiate buildup of plaque in arteries, suppress the immune system, cause digestive disorders, and damage the reproductive organs and lungs.

- Clean up your gut. Keeping the ecosystem in your intestinal tract healthy and balanced will keep you regular and fight against low-grade infections (including yeast infections), food allergies, and other gastrointestinal ailments.
- Drink lots and lots of clean, filtered water. Nothing dilutes poisons and cleans like good old H_2O.

GMOS=OMG!

Topping the ever-growing list of things to do to protect our health: steering clear of genetically modified organisms (GMOs). A GMO is an organism—plant, bacteria, animal—that has had its genetic structure artificially engineered, or modified, to create a different organism. For example, a particular type of corn may be engineered to resist diseases or to guarantee larger yields. Much of our food is being messed with in laboratories, and the result is what I like to think of as an agricultural "hate child" of modern technology merging with corporate greed. Big biotech companies do not have your best interests at heart. I don't know about you, but patenting the world's food supply doesn't sound like such a good idea to me.

Some companies have also contractually limited farmers' ability to use GM seeds from their crops. Farmers must buy new seeds every year instead of growing from the previous year's yield. Ironically, GM crops have shown no increase in yield. GMOs are bad for your body, bad for the community, bad for farmers, and bad for the environment. Here are some compelling reasons why you should avoid GMOs:

- We don't know the long-term health outcomes of consuming GM foods. GM plants, such as soybean, corn, cottonseed, and canola, have had foreign genes forced into their DNA. The inserted genes come from species, such as bacteria and viruses, that have never been in the human food supply. Genetic engineering transfers genes across natural species barriers. It uses imprecise laboratory techniques that bear no resemblance to natural breeding and are based on outdated concepts of how genes and cells work. Gene insertion is done either by shooting genes from a "gene gun" into a plate of cells or by using bacteria to invade the cell with foreign DNA. The altered cell is then cloned into a plant. It is unknown how these new strains of bacteria may affect our body systems' balance.

- As I write this, foods that contain GMOs are not labeled in the United States. Americans already have a tough time deciphering claims on nutrition labels and breaking down the nutritional status of a food. So if your labels aren't showing you what ingredients lie within, the margin of opportunity to eat clean foods diminishes. Several states are working to pass legislation mandating that GMO foods must be labeled as such, but large conglomerates invested in GMOs spend enormous amounts of money to defeat such attempts. The European Union has banned GMOs, as have Australia, Japan, and two dozen other countries. These countries recognize that a lack of long-term studies and testing may be hiding disastrous health defects.

Here in the United States, the House of Representatives 2013 Agriculture Appropriations Bill contained a provision, dubbed by some as the "Monsanto Protection Act," that gives the agriculture biotech industry the ability to get temporary

USDA approval or deregulation of a GM crop, even if the safety of the crop is under challenge. The passage of this provision has been met with public outcry and several members of Congress have pledged not to extend it when the bill comes up for renewal. Only time will tell.

· Genetic engineering reduces genetic diversity. This pretty much tosses the evolutionary concept "survival of the fittest" right out the window. When genes are more diverse, they are naturally more robust, which is why purebred animals have more health problems than mixed breeds. Plants with reduced genetic diversity cannot handle drought, fungus invasions, or insects as well as natural plants can. That can have dire consequences for farmers and communities.

· Studies conducted on GM foods don't look so hot. Thousands of sheep, buffaloes, and goats in India died after grazing on GMO cotton plants following harvest. Others suffered poor health and reproductive problems. Farmers in Europe and Asia say that cows, water buffaloes, chickens, and horses died from eating GMO corn varieties. About two dozen US farmers report that GMO corn varieties caused widespread sterility in pigs and cows.

Simple Tips to Avoiding GMOs

1. Purchase certified organic foods that are GMO-free, and tell your friends and loved ones to do the same.
2. Download your free *Non-GMO Shopping Guide* or Apple's ShopNoGMO iPhone app and use it when you go food shopping. This is published by the Institute for Responsible Technology (IRT) and founded by activist and author Jeffrey Smith to educate policy makers and the public about GMOs.
3. Read the books *Seeds of Change* and *Genetic Roulette: The Documented Health Risks of Genetically Engineered Foods* by Jeffrey Smith.

4. Sign petitions against GMOs at Food Democracy Now!
   (www.fooddemocracynow.org). FDN is a grassroots
   movement of over 650,000 farmers and citizens dedicated
   to building a sustainable food system that gives our
   communities access to healthy foods and respects the
   dignity of the farmers who produce those foods.
5. Steer clear of all processed foods, as well as nonorganic
   soy, rice, papaya, tomatoes, rapeseed, dairy, potatoes,
   peas, corn, and conventionally farmed meats, to limit your
   exposure to GMOs.

Lastly, don't underestimate the power of exercise in the fight against toxins. When we work up a sweat, we release all kinds of beneficial chemicals into our bloodstreams, while the body purges unwanted substances via perspiration. Working out also reminds us to hydrate well.

We can take a positive page from our cavewomen sisters by emulating their chemical-free lifestyles to the best of our ability. Keeping it green, whole, and fresh goes a long way toward giving our bodies a fighting chance in getting our gorgeous groove back.

CHAPTER 5

Good Carbs, Bad Carbs

or the past twenty-five years, it has been hammered into us, by one fad diet or another, that we have to cut carbs entirely from our diets in order to lose weight. So we immediately stop eating anything with carbs. We lose some weight, thinking, *Hey, this isn't so bad.* Then within a couple of weeks, we realize we're *starving* and could lick the food in magazine ads. We think, *One small baked potato, a few slices of a baguette, and a scoop of dulce de leche ice cream every so often won't hurt.* Before long, it's *Oh, what the hell! I'd rather be fat and sated than skinny and starving.* We're off to the races again. Our hunger is sated, and our jeans don't fit. They're even tighter than before we stopped eating carbs. So what gives?

Here's what gives: we have become utterly confused—and misled—about how and why carbohydrates are a must-have in our diets.

Let's start with the basics. Carbohydrates provide the nutrients we need to fuel our bodies. We need the energy locked up in carbs (which the body converts to glucose) to build muscle, keep our nervous systems in fine form, build and maintain our cells, and balance our hormones. There are three basic types of carbs. Because of—yet again—the marketing muscle of food manufacturers—we get all tied up in knots when we try to make sense of which carbs are good for us and which are bad. I'm going to make understanding all of this as easy as pie.

1. Simple Carbohydrates. These are carbs that are, literally, made up only of sugars (usually just one or two), and these are the carbs that we need to avoid. Ingesting simple carbs is like mainlining glucose: so much is swept into our bloodstreams that our insulin levels spike. These "foods" (if you can call them that) are the ones that cause that "sugar rush" feeling. You know, you haven't eaten for hours, so you have a slice of cake at the office birthday party or stop for a doughnut. Shortly after eating said cake or doughnut, you get a sudden surge of energy—and then, within an hour or two, you come crashing down. This kind of fast delivery of glucose shocks our systems—and so our metabolisms—and makes us fat.

Culprits include pasta, bread, and baked goods made with white flour; anything with table sugar, fruit juice, corn syrup, and jam; and packaged cereals. (This is why you *have* to read those nutrition and ingredient labels!)

So when it comes to carbs, avoid the simple ones. Because what they will do to your metabolism is anything but.

2. Complex Carbohydrates. Our bodies (and minds) love complex carbs. Yes, they contain sugars, but they also have fiber, which means that it take much longer and is much harder—more complex—for the body to break down and absorb. Since complex carbs take longer to digest and absorb, they provide a slow, steady stream of energy. Our insulin levels remain consistent, and we stay satisfied and sharp. And this is a beautiful thing.

For Paleo Chic purposes, you'll find complex carbs in dark leafy greens, fruits, cruciferous vegetables, and other nutritious foods.

But here's the rub with complex carbs. Before the industrial revolution (pre-1900), Americans ate a ton of complex carbs but were not, as a society, obese, which just goes to show what creating food in a factory, as opposed to on a farm, does in terms of wrecking the health benefits of that food. The fattening-food industrial complex has taken our Paleo carbs and mixed them with refined sugars and all sorts of other chemicals, boxed them up, and has the cojones to sell these Frankenfoods to us as healthy carbs. This is where we need to put on our big-girl Paleo panties and say "Enough is enough!"

3. Indigestible Carbohydrates. These carbohydrates, also known as dietary fiber, are so dense and indigestible that they don't offer any significant energy to our bodies. They do, however, provide the necessary roughage to keep our digestive wheels turning so that when the next healthy carb comes through, our bodies can take what they need and eliminate the rest. Do your body justice with nuts, ground flaxseeds, and fresh fruits and vegetables such as apples and broccoli. Keep things fresh and enjoy them raw, cooked, and juiced.

Why Cavewomen Don't Do Uber-Low Carb

When we go all crazy and cut out too many carbs, we run the risk of starving our bodies of necessary energy in ways that cause a domino effect of maladaptive metabolic processes. Without sufficient amounts of the right kind of sugar for fuel, our bodies have to work to convert other nutrients, such as protein, into energy. This is like stealing from Peter in order to pay Paul: if protein is hijacked for fuel, then it's not available to make new cells or regulate our hormones. If we're starved of most carbs, our bodies can't metabolize fat properly (fats need components of carbs to break down, ladies), and we generate ketones, a by-product of out-of-whack fat conversion. We get fooled when our bodies go into this "shock" state, because ketosis tamps down our appetites. When we're in a severely low-carb state, we run the risk of becoming dehydrated, our brains go all mushy, and our muscles (which are now being broken down for fuel) weaken. So, yes, we may drop a few pounds temporarily, but with them goes our ability to think and move well.

So what's a cavewoman to do? The easiest way to figure out how to manage the three kinds of carbs (simple, complex, and indigestible) is to follow these three rules:

1. Eat lots and lots of naturally occurring complex carbs. These include all fresh fruits and vegetables, sweet potatoes, winter squash, jicamas, taros, and Jerusalem artichokes.
2. Scale back your intake of fruit juices, as well as refined and highly processed flour products. That's just about anything you can buy in a box or a bag: cookies, chips, crackers, breads, premixed convenience foods, and so forth.
3. Banish sugars (refined and unrefined), syrups, jams, jellies, and any item that has simple sugars added to it.

Sugar: The Necessary Evil

Since our bodies basically run on sugars—metabolically converted sugars—why is eating sugar so bad for us?

Because sugar is corrosive in the extreme. And we're literally choking ourselves on this stuff. In 2012 the US Department of Agriculture estimated that Americans consume roughly forty-seven pounds of sugar and thirty-five pounds of high-fructose corn syrup every year. That's more than eighty pounds *per person* per year of raw, fattening fuel! This statistic alone ought to be enough to scare you straight about sugar, but if not, I'll keep going.

Over the past thirty years, Americans have been diagnosed with type 2 diabetes, hypertension, heart disease, and cancers at accelerated rates never seen before. And our overconsumption of sugars can play a role in all of these diseases.

The Lure of Those White Lines

Who knew that your local grocery store is really a cover for a very sinister, postmodern version of Studio 54? Every time you pull a box of some sugar-drenched product off the shelf, you might as well be back in the glory days of disco, hunched over in a dark corner, snorting lines of the white stuff. This may sound like a preposterous analogy, but it's not, because sugar is as addictive as crack cocaine. (It trips the same dopamine receptors in the pleasure parts of our brains.) Our bodies and brains aren't naturally hard-wired to need this form of sugar, but once we get it, we just can't get enough. Once we flip that switch, we slide down a sweet, slippery slope, and there's just no "off" setting. When it comes to pleasure and our brains, we want more and more sugar!

So stay away from the white stuff and watch out for refined sugar's evil twin, high-fructose corn syrup, which the food industry has managed to put into just about everything. Fructose is the worst of the worst. And HFCS is even more harmful. Food giants in agribusiness are now actually trying to promote refined sugar as "good." They're slapping the words "Contains No High-Fructose Corn Syrup" on their products to make us think that their products are healthy. In an effort to increase the bottom line, these companies substitute one destructive type of unhealthy sugar for another. Who would've ever thought that white sugar would rise up to be the "good" girl? It's all relative, isn't it!

Fructose is not—I repeat, not—glucose. And it's not your body's friend. Let me break it down a bit: refined white sugar (sucrose) contains a 50–50 mixture of glucose and fructose. HFCS contains 55 percent fructose and 45 percent glucose. Only the liver metabolizes the fructose component of sugar and HFCS, but every cell in the body metabolizes the glucose from sugar and starches. Fructose puts a huge metabolic burden on your liver, but glucose requires only 20 percent participation from that organ. When too much fructose enters the liver, the body cannot process it quickly enough.

Fructose ravages your metabolic system and wreaks havoc on your endocrine system, liver, and vascular system. Drinking sodas or high-fructose drinks (sports drinks are the worst) is like shooting up poison: your liver pretty much goes into shock with every can of the stuff you knock back.

Here's what else fructose does to you:

- For every 120 calories of fructose that you consume, your body stores 40 of those as fat. Compare this with eating 120 calories of glucose: your body hangs on to less than 1 calorie of fat.
- When your liver goes into fructose shock, it overproduces uric acid, which, in turn, leads to high blood pressure and inflammation. (The severe joint pain known as gout, caused by excess uric acid in the blood, is common in those who overdose on fructose.)
- Eating fructose triggers insulin resistance, which means that fat droplets get dispersed into your muscles, your liver, and your other vital organs. Insulin resistance is early-stage type 2 diabetes, the gateway disease to all kinds of health woes.
- Your body needs glucose. When it gets fructose instead, it goes into fat-producing mode rather than fat-burning mode.
- Research shows that ingesting fructose hampers brain functioning and dulls synaptic signaling. This, in turn, warps our ability to learn and muddles our memory. Perhaps this is one explanation for the rise in diagnoses of attention deficit/ hyperactivity disorder (ADHD) and other brain-related conditions in our kids. Research also indicates that fructose overload may contribute to Alzheimer's disease.
- Fructose causes systemic inflammation, which can lead to autoimmune diseases, including arthritis, heart disease, and, of course, obesity.

Probably the greatest challenge on the Paleo Chic plan is eliminating sugar from your diet. I will not sugarcoat how hard it is stop eating sugar: our dependence on sugar is a physiological addiction. Quitting cold turkey rarely works. Your goal is to simultaneously taper off sugar while eating more protein and fat, so your body can quickly experience how energized, clean, and lean it feels when it's not being polluted with all that unhealthy sweet stuff.

When we overindulge in carbs and sugars, we don't allow our bodies to metabolize (and burn) fats the way they want to. The plain truth is, our bodies can process only so many carbs, and they have very limited ways, other than producing fat, to store excesses of this nutrient. That's why, as we age, we tend to develop a muffin top around our middle—this is the body's way of telling us that we're eating too many carbs.

Keeping Your Insulin Level Low

Sugar also does a serious number on our blood sugar levels. When our blood is saturated with too much sugar, all kinds of things go wrong. Most alarmingly, our insulin levels are called upon to be too high, too much of the time, and this, in turn, teaches our bodies not to respond to the hormone (the phenomenon known as insulin resistance). Here's what happens when there's too much insulin coursing through our systems:

- Elevated insulin levels suppress production of the hormones glucagon and GH. Glucagon takes stored fat and breaks it down into sugar, while growth hormone is needed to create lean muscle mass.
- High insulin levels mess with your appetite. Ever indulge in a huge bowl of pasta at a late dinner and then wake up the next morning to find your stomach growling with hunger? This occurs because that high-carb meal gave you a spike of sugars rather than a steady delivery of fuel.

- Too much insulin compromises the body's ability to dismantle fat. It doesn't matter how much time you spend on that treadmill. If you're eating too much sugar, your body is going to fight and hold on to any unwanted fat for dear life.

That's why you have to eliminate all of the unhealthy carbs from your diet and make a point of loading up on healthy carbs. It's that simple—and that challenging.

To become a bad-carbs private dick, you have to read every label before you put any food in your grocery cart.

CARBOHYDRATES: RULES TO LIVE BY

1. A gram of carbohydrates has 4 calories and a gram of protein has 4 calories, but the body metabolizes them in entirely different ways. Carbohydrates are isocaloric but not isometabolic, while proteins are isocaloric and isometabolic. This means that you can eat 100 calories from steak, chicken, or eggs, and they will all have the exact same effect on your body. But if you eat 100 calories of glucose from a potato or bread or 100 calories of sugar (half glucose and half fructose), they will be metabolized differently and have a different effect on your body. A calorie isn't just a calorie when the metabolic consequences are completely different.

2. Carbohydrates raise insulin and cortisol, the fat-storage hormones, for up to five hours after ingestion. Protein typically has a negligible effect on insulin levels. If you eat an excess of protein with too little dietary fat, then you may wind up with elevated blood glucose. This is rarely the case, but let's put it out there so that all the bases are covered.

3. You will burn far more body fat and lose more weight if you replace carbohydrates with protein, calorie for calorie. This means that if two people are eating an 1,800-calorie diet, the one eating 15 percent protein will store more fat than

the one eating 25 percent protein, which will burn more fat. Low-carbohydrate, high-protein diets reduce weight more effectively after six months than low-fat diets do after one year. No more yo-yo dieting for you!

Protein and fat are the dominatrixes of the brain; carbohydrates are its bitch. Protein and fat regulate brain biochemistry and appetite control through the proper production of neurotransmitters; carbohydrates can wreak havoc on this delicate balance. We've been brainwashed to believe that fat is the enemy, while processed carbohydrates are the good guys; this doesn't make physiological sense.

4. There have been many studies about what time of day is best to eat your carbs. Assuming you eat carbs daily, this can vary based on how you feel and how you burn fat. After a workout, some people like to have a protein shake with fruit and then eat carbs at their next full meal. Others like to eat their carbs at night because they feel carbs help them sleep better. Experiment to see what works best for you. If you don't eat any starches at all, or eat starches only on the days that you work out, then keep on rocking!

Counting Grams of Sugar

When I ask my clients if they overindulge in sugar, most of them swear that they don't. But when I ask them to grab pen and paper and do a quick sugar gram inventory based on what's in their pantries and fridges, they go into shock. That's because sugar likes to hide out in unlikely places, such as a container of "fat-free" yogurt, a protein bar, "low-fat" granola, and low-cal energy drinks. I would go so far as to say that whenever you see the words *low calorie, fat-free,* or *healthy* on a package, it's a tip-off that it's loaded with sugar.

Your job is to become a sugar detective and call it out whenever and wherever you find it. And banish it from your kitchen. You need to know what a gram of sugar is and approach each gram of sugar as though it were a gram of a highly toxic substance.

WHAT'S IN A GRAM OF SUGAR?

Here's the big takeaway: 1 teaspoon of sugar is equal to 4 grams of sugar. Memorize that. Drill it into your brain. Never forget it. If you're going to eat foods that contain sugars, you need to limit your intake to 4 grams (or 1 teaspoon) per serving. You heard right: 4 grams. Of sugar. Per serving.

Most fruit juices and sodas have anywhere from 10 to 12 teaspoons (40 to 48 grams) of sugar per 8 ounces. This means that drinking just one "serving" means you're getting 10 servings worth of sugar. Minimum. Given that the American Heart Association has set a daily intake limit for sugar at 30 grams per day (too generous), that means you've overshot your daily allotment in just a few gulps. Those 30 grams of sugar—a whopping 7.5 teaspoons—is roughly 120 calories of sugar. At this maximum baseline, eating this much sugar means that you're ingesting roughly 850 calories a week in sugar alone. For my Paleo Chic clients, striving to stay at or below this level reflects either (at the beginning of the plan) a massive reduction in their sugar intake or that they're pretty much right on target.

Cavewomen are encouraged to substitute healthy proteins or fat choices in place of sweets. If you do, you will watch your sweet tooth disappear as you watch the pounds melt away. You can take that to the bank.

How to Subdue Your Sweet Cravings

There are things you can do—right now—to help wean yourself off sugar.

- Eat a protein-dense breakfast that features some healthful fats. This will superload your metabolism with slow-burning fuels and will keep your blood sugar levels steady. I'm a big believer in eating dinner for breakfast. (I bet that any self-respecting cavewoman started her day with some meat or fish and a salad.) Enjoy an egg, a lamb chop, or some shrimp in the morning, and toss in a handful of nuts while you're at it. Don't be surprised if you no longer experience a midafternoon crash.

- Whenever you crave something sweet, opt for a blood-sugar-stabilizing protein and/or fat instead. Skip the low-fat yogurt and have some turkey slices rolled up with avocado, or some apple slices smeared with almond butter. When you choose a healthy alternative, your cravings for sugar will retreat. One of my favorite sugar busters is a steaming cuppa hot cocoa: add 1 tablespoon of cocoa powder to 8 ounces boiling water and top with a dash of cinnamon.

- Check in with your level of thirst. Often, we think we're hungry when we're actually thirsty, and this is when we tend to snack on things that aren't good for us. Instead, immediately have a tall, cool glass of water with a squeeze of lemon. Then wait a few minutes. If you're still not satisfied, enjoy a cup of naturally flavored tea. (I like cinnamon or licorice root.) Or chill out with an iced hot chocolate: dissolve 1 tablespoon organic cocoa powder in 8 ounces hot water. Pour over a tall glass of ice and enjoy some liquid love.

- Lastly, there's always the power of chocolate. Eating chocolate with a higher cocoa content is a natural mood booster. If we increase those feel-good neurotransmitters, we not only give our brain biochemistry a shot in the arm but also stop our cravings in their tracks. So if you need to throw a bone at your dopamine receptors, have a square of organic dark chocolate that's at least 70 percent cacao.

WHAT ABOUT NATURALLY OCCURRING SUGARS?

Many of my clients operate under the assumption that nature-made sugars such as honey and maple syrup are somehow "better" for them than refined sugars. These sugars are metabolized by the body in the exact same way as their manufactured counterparts, so they're not part of the Paleo Chic plan. That said, eating honey, especially if raw and unpasteurized, and maple syrup in minimal amounts is preferable, because they offer other (albeit tiny) nutritional benefits.

WHAT'S THE DEAL WITH SUGAR SUBSTITUTES?

We all have to make responsible choices when living life Paleo Chic, since all of these sweeteners act the same way in the body as sugar, so here are some options.

If there's a sweetener that's Paleo friendly, it's honey. Raw honey is a completely unprocessed food; no other sweetener can hold that claim. Even maple syrup and molasses require some processing before they're ready to eat. Biochemically speaking, honey is made up of 40 percent glucose, 36 percent fructose, and 24 percent other sugars. This can vary, depending on what the bees have been eating, but you get the general idea.

Maple syrup is relatively low in fructose and contains the trace minerals manganese, potassium, iron, and calcium. Molasses is basically table sugar, but with a splash of nutrition; it contains iron, calcium, and magnesium. Coconut palm sugar is relatively new to the scene, but it is rich in magnesium, nitrogen, and vitamin C. Agave is the prom queen of natural sweeteners, and I hailed its merits in my earlier books. But don't be fooled: agave also contains 90 percent fructose and the toxic compound saponins. So steer clear of agave—it's a wolf in sheep's clothing.

Trace minerals notwithstanding, think of these natural sweeteners in the context of a good-better-best scenario. Yes, they're more nutritious than sugar, but you still need to consume them judiciously. Every cavewoman knows that sweeteners are not accessible in nature in the same quantities as the aisles of the grocery store. Honey is well protected by bees and hard to access in nature. And cavewomen certainly did not troll maple trees with spigots in hand to tap the syrup. So bear this in mind when having a Paleo-style treat or cheat meal; once a week should do the trick!

WHAT ABOUT SYNTHETIC SWEETENERS?

Do you think any self-respecting cavewoman whipped out a small pink or blue packet when she wanted a sweet treat and dumped it on her food? Synthetic sweeteners are nothing more than glammed-up garbage and contain some pretty scandalous chemicals. Although they are marketed as being natural, they're anything but. In fact, there's a lot of controversy surrounding the potential hazards of artificial sweeteners—enough to raise an eyebrow or two. Aspartame, acesulfame potassium (also known as acesulfame K), neotame, saccharin, and sucralose are all linked to significant health concerns, despite being approved by the US Food and Drug Administration (FDA). Words such as *neurotoxicity, formaldehyde,* and *chlorinated* are all part of the synthetic sweetener vocabulary. I don't know about you, but I'm outta here!

One more thing I should mention: contrary to the word *diet*, these fake foods will not help you lose weight. There's enough research out there showing that diet soda drinkers wind up with larger waist circumferences and higher fasting glucose levels to disprove the belief that you won't get fat drinking diet sodas. Although you may know you're chugging an aspartame-sweetened soda, your body may not. The sweet flavor tickling your taste buds will trick your brain into thinking that you've treated your body to something sweet and delicious, and your pancreas will pour out insulin in response. Kiss *buh-bye* any fat burning that your body is doing. Is the risk worth it? No way, José!

If you really want to be the lean, mean, fun-loving machine you deserve to be, there's just no way around it: you have to take sugar— in all of its refined glory—out of your life, along with synthetic sweeteners. When you do so, your head and skin will miraculously clear up, you'll slim down, and you'll build lean muscle mass. You will feel balanced and clean and whole in a way that sugar just can't touch.

SUGAR ALCOHOLS: BETTER OPTIONS?

Sugar alcohols definitely do not fall within the Paleo realm of eating, but the reality is that low-carb lovers use them regularly, so it warrants a discussion about the impact they can have on your body. If you haven't previously used them, I wouldn't tell you to run out and start now, but if you are using them, here's what you need to know.

Sugar alcohols can be found in sugar-free products such as protein bars and sugar-free candy. They're neither sugar nor an alcohol. So what do they do inside your body?

Sugar alcohols occur naturally in plants. Sorbitol is derived from corn syrup; maltitol is derived from seaweed. Mostly, though, they are made from sugars and starches. Although sugar alcohols are similar to sugar, they are not completely absorbed by the body. They have fewer calories than sugar and can actually help fight tooth decay. Xylitol is now added to toothpastes and chewing gum for this very reason.

What are the downsides to sugar alcohols? To sum up things quite succinctly: farting. Quickly followed by bloating and/or diarrhea. And, like the artificial sweeteners, they too can have a glycemic effect on your blood sugar. Mannitol is the worst offender, here. Erythritol seems to have the most inconsequential effects on blood sugar, but if your body doesn't process sugar alcohols well, you're still going to drop some nasty bombs.

Stevia isn't without controversy, but it seems to be the best of the sugar substitutes. *Stevia rebaundiana* is an herb from South America that is dried and refined into a sweet powder or liquid. Stevia is three hundred times sweeter than sugar, has a negligible amount of calories, and—my favorite part—exerts a negligible effect on blood sugar levels. There are no toxic side effects to stevia, which is why it is the only sweetener I recommend on a regular basis. It can be used in smoothies, cooking, baking, and hot beverages. I use a pinch of stevia in a cup of hot cocoa and up to ¼ cup to replace sugar in a baked goods recipe. The flavor difference is subtle, and you can still satisfy your sweet tooth without the metabolic consequences of sugar.

SUGAR BY ANY OTHER NAME

Food manufacturers are deceptive when it comes to listing ingredients on labels. They bank on the fact that as long as something tastes good, you'll keep buying it. And when products are laced with sugar, you become hooked faster and become a repeat customer. Beware! All of the following ingredients are just other names for sugar. You don't need to memorize this list, but the more familiar you become with these names, the faster you'll recognize them as giant red flags that will make you fat and keep you there! I've also included some sugar alcohols (any word ending in -*ol*) because they are used as sweeteners in reduced-calorie and low-calorie foods. And one more thing: even if a product is labeled organic, it's still sugar and will still have the same metabolic consequences as sugar.

Agave nectar	Carob syrup	Corn syrup solids
Barley malt	Castor sugar	Crystalline
Beet sugar	Coconut palm	fructose
Brown rice syrup	sugar	Date sugar
Cane crystals	Confectioners'	Dextran
Cane juice crystals	sugar	Dextrose
Cane sugar	Corn sweetener	Diastatic malt
Caramel	Corn syrup	Diatase

Ethyl maltol	High-fructose corn	Maple syrup
Evaporated cane	syrup	Molasses
juice	Honey	Muscovado sugar
Fructose	Hydrogenated	Panocha
Fruit juice	starch	Raw sugar
Fruit juice	hydrolysates	Refiners' syrup
concentrates	Invert sugar	Rice syrup
Galactose	Isomalt	Sorbitol
Glucose	Lactose	Sorghum syrup
Glucose solids	Malt syrup	Sucanat
Golden sugar	Maltitol	Sucrose
Golden syrup	Maltodextrin	Syrup
Granulated sugar	Maltose	Turbinado sugar
Grape sugar	Mannitol	

Where Did That Muffin Top Come From?

We humans have been ingesting cultivated grains for only about ten thousand years, which is just a tiny blip on the human timeline. (We managed to get by as hunter-gatherers for two hundred thousand years before then.) Our appetites for cultivated grains grew as we discovered and adopted better farming practices, not an entirely good thing.

And here is why: our brains and bodies are designed to function best when they're fueled largely by proteins and fats. Yes, yes, we need the nutrients provided by carbohydrates for optimal health, but it's all a question of balance, and as we moved into an agricultural way of life, we began to tip the dietary balance in favor of carbs over proteins and fats. Ten thousand years later, we find ourselves eating a diet that is deleteriously dense in carbs. Couple this change in the way we eat with the fact that we no longer chase after our food. What's happened is the double whammy of becoming way more sedentary than our ancestors and eating fat-creating foods rather than speed- and muscle-building foods.

What's a Paleo Chic girl to do?

Giving up grains is the only way.

How can this possibly be when we're bombarded with messages such as "Eat a bowl of this high-fiber, high-energy cereal every morning, and you will slim down!" This approach—telling people to eat more carbs—drives me nuts. Eating grains triggers your brain to want more empty carbs, and that creates a vicious cycle of over-eating the wrong nutrient sources. And this, ladies, is precisely what makes and keeps us fat.

Giving Up Grains

Probably the most controversial aspect of the Paleo Chic diet is that I advocate cutting out all grains. (And you thought you'd just have to give up sweets!) Yes, you heard right: if you're going to really eat like a cavewoman, you have let go of all of the neocarbs. Neocarbs are postagricultural carbs and include all mass-cultivated grains, such as wheat, corn, oats, and rye. We're in an age when we're confronted with a host of illnesses that are the direct result of our love affair with neocarbs, and these include gluten intolerance, Celiac disease, and, of course, obesity.

Our cavewoman ancestors were hunter-gatherers, and so the carbs they ate—the true Paleocarbs—included fruits and vegetables that grew seasonally and in the wild, as well as roots and tubers. Modern-day equivalents include yams, sweet potatoes, squashes, jicamas, and Jerusalem artichokes, to name just a few. Once you try them, you'll see how satisfying and delicious they are.

It's not easy to give grains and gluten the old heave-ho, especially if you've been eating them all your life. Let's face it: grains taste good and have long been some of our favorite comfort foods.

But if you're ready to make significant changes in how you eat and how you look, then they have to go. I know how hard this can be. I've been there. It took me years to reach where I am now, because I wasn't emotionally or physically ready for it in my twenties. Start by making small adjustments. Have a Paleo breakfast every day, eat greens at every meal, or skip the sweets for one week. You will soon feel better, and that will keep you on the path to Paleo Chic.

Back in the early days of growing grains, farmers harvested grains mellowed in the fields for several weeks before they were threshed and beaten to separate the grains and seeds from the stalks. This gave the seeds time to sprout and even ferment, which reduced the phytic acid content and made the grains easier to digest. Nowadays, grains are grown using crazy steroid-like, biologically engineered methodologies (Would you like some delicious genetic modification with your bread, popcorn, or rice?), and as soon as they're "ready" (whatever that means), they're harvested, sent into whatever high-processing factory they're destined for, sprinkled with chemical fairy dust (sugars, preservatives), and boxed up in pretty packages that we find irresistible.

But with all of this dazzling advancement has come our greatest and most far-reaching health woes. Going Paleo, pushing past all of those glitzy grains, will lead you out of the food wilderness, and you'll find yourself standing on a verdant plain, feeling your absolute best.

Gluten: Go With Your Gut

Gluten is the protein found in wheat and other grains that is essential for the process of leavening. (Leavening is when the gases held within grains are released and lets dough ferment.) Gluten breaks down the microvilli that line our guts and allow for the efficient absorption of food in the small intestine. When these fingerlike projections become damaged or destroyed, we experience uncomfortable and distressing symptoms such as bloating, gas, pain, constipation, and diarrhea. If the damage is severe, we might succumb to a condition called "leaky gut syndrome," which is when the contents of the intestines—food particles and toxins—actually leak out of the bowel and into our bloodstream. This can then trigger a host of autoimmune conditions. (When under siege like this, our body will go into "fight" mode and will try to rid itself of these irritants.) Other autoimmune diseases exacerbated by gluten consumption are Crohn's disease, lupus, and multiple sclerosis. Studies show that cutting gluten from the diet lessens the severity of these very serious conditions.

Lectin: Gluten's Sidekick

Lectins, tiny proteins that are ubiquitous in nature (yup, they're inside of all of us), are found in all plants, particularly legumes, as well as in animals. These sugar- (carb-) binding, potent fungicides protect seeds from molds and insects. Think about that for a moment: lectins are basically naturally occurring pesticides. When we eat foods that are high in lectins, we are, in essence, eating a toxin, and lectin overload aggravates a number of health problems, including Crohn's, colitis, irritable bowel syndrome, Hashimoto's thyroiditis, fibromyalgia, chronic fatigue syndrome, and arthritis. Ingesting too much lectin can also cause depression, as serotonin is actually secreted in the intestines.

Most globally, lectin contributes to weight gain by disrupting the body's ability to break down and metabolize glucose. (Remember, lectin is a sugar-seeking protein.) When this happens, the hormone insulin can't do its job and, once again, we pack on the pounds.

Lectin also blocks the healthy flow of digestive hormones and makes metabolizing lectin-rich foods (legumes, soy, green peas, corn, potatoes, and especially wheat germ) tricky. Lectins can increase our appetite, make us feel bloated and out of whack, and mess with the body's ability to extract nutrients efficiently. That's why any weight-loss program that even suggests a moderate to high amount of carbohydrates (especially modern grains) will set you up for failure.

The double-whammy of gluten and lectin intolerances leaves many feeling fatigued, fat, and out of sorts. Although there are tests for gluten and lectin intolerance, I suggest to my clients that they just give these foods a rest for a month or so and see how they feel. Many see and feel remarkable changes: increased regularity, less bloating and gas, and a feeling of being sated and even-keeled in such a short amount of time. They quickly get the message of how invasive and annoying gluten and lectins are.

Here is a quick hit-list of high-gluten, high-lectin foods to avoid:

Amaranth	Oats
Barley	Rye
Beans and legumes	Quinoa
Corn	Soy
High-fructose corn syrup	Spelt
Kamut	Wheat
Millet	

Instead, stock your cave with these gluten-free, lectin-free Paleo Chic carbs:

Leafy green (especially dark) vegetables
Jerusalem artichokes
Jicamas
Low-sugar fruits: berries, peaches, plums, apricots, oranges,
    plantains, grapefruits, apples, pears, cantaloupes
Shirataki mushroom pasta
Spaghetti squash

Sweet potatoes or yams
Taros
Winter squashes

If you can make the leap and go all-out Paleo for just one month, I can guarantee that you'll get such an amazing glimpse at your glamorous, irresistible new self that you will never, ever want to go back to your old way of eating.

CHAPTER 6

Paleo Chic Women Love Meat

Here's the nitty-gritty on the Paleo Chic plan: protein is the new superfood. You heard right: protein is the mother of all macronutrients when it comes to being lean, strong, and healthy.

I have no clue why my very savvy, smart clients have a lot of resistance to eating protein—especially to eating meat.

I hear all kinds of crazy, messed-up thinking when it comes to why women shy away from eating more protein, including things such as:

"Won't eating protein bulk me up?" Actually, sweetheart, eating protein will slim you down.

"Doesn't red meat cause cancer and heart disease?" Actually, eating grass-fed, hormone-free beef can provide your body with necessary nutrients that can help to prevent heart disease and certain cancers.

"Won't I be hungry if I eat more meat and cut back on my carbs?" This is the one that drives me crazy because it's protein—*protein*—that best satisfies us and eliminates hunger.

The Power of Protein

Proteins are, quite literally, the building blocks of life. They are made up of long chains of amino acids. Dietary protein, found in meat, eggs, poultry, and fish, is essential for the body to function, because we don't produce all the amino acids we need and must ingest them.

Proteins make up a big part of who we are. Nearly 50 percent of our "dry" cell weight is protein. It plays a key role in so many of our vital metabolic processes, such as digestion, heart health (protein builds the heart muscle!), and muscle and cell regeneration—all of the things that make us strong, fit, and vital.

The beauty of protein as a nutritional superfood is its slow delivery. Proteins don't shock or overtax our systems the way carbs do. Instead, they immediately go to work by triggering the production of hormones that release key digestive enzymes, providing a sense of satiety, and working to restore cellular health.

Protein: Why We Need More, More, More

Most forms of protein aren't convenience foods that you can toss into your handbag, but, calorie for calorie, protein packs a huge wallop in comparison to the same number of calories you'd get in carbohydrates. For instance, 6 ounces of salmon can have the same calories as a large chocolate chip cookie, but the metabolic consequences are entirely different.

How much protein should you eat every day? A good formula is to aim for at least 1 ounce per pound of body weight. So if you weigh 150 pounds, eat 150 grams of protein a day. There are 7 grams of protein in an ounce, so 150 grams of protein equals 21 ounces per day. This means that you can eat an average of 5 ounces at meals, and another 2 to 3 ounces for each snack.

A slew of recent studies shows that most women ages eighteen to forty-five (a good chunk of the population, in other words) aren't eating the recommended daily minimum of protein in their diets.

What?

You heard right. The US Department of Agriculture suggests conservatively that every woman's diet should include at least 10 percent to 15 percent of lean protein. That's far less than the 25 percent that many health organizations recommend. Studies have found that a diet consisting of 25 percent lean protein will lower blood pressure, improve cholesterol and triglyceride (fats in the blood) levels, and will boost key levels of nutrients such as iron, vitamin D, and calcium in women, thereby protecting us from oste-oporosis (bone density loss), diabetes, and other diseases. Oh, and a high-protein diet also helps us lose weight.

And contrary to some popular myths, protein is not difficult on our systems. The minute that protein hits your tongue, it starts to work its magic by spreading the message throughout your body that it is being well fed and that all "starvation" concerns are now being addressed. Your metabolism begins to work optimally when you ingest protein—including your fat-burning processes!

Studies also show that making protein up to 30 percent of our daily intake means that we eat, on average, 450 fewer calories a day. This kind of radical reduction in calorie intake can lead to pretty dramatic weight loss—in the range of, say, a pound a week. And this is without making any other significant lifestyle changes. (No added exercise, no other dietary tweaks.) Now we're cooking with gas!

These studies also show that front-loading the day with a big dose of protein at breakfast (think 4 to 5 ounces) is the best way to jump-start those weight-shedding mechanisms. Eating animal protein for breakfast also does wonders for your blood sugar lev-els. Once you start eating some meat, fish, or poultry to break that overnight fast, that three-in-the-afternoon energy crash becomes a thing of the past.

Not all proteins carry the desired amino acid punch your body needs. Just as there are good carbs and bad carbs, some proteins are better for you than others. Our Paleo ancestors were onto something when they opted for meat over, say, legumes, because not all plant-based proteins carry the nine amino acids our bodies need to produce lean muscle. Believe it or not, the most ab-friendly, belly-busting proteins are flesh proteins: pastured poultry, wild seafood, and grass-fed meats.

How Protein Balances Brain Biochemistry

Eating protein sends a strong signal to your brain's hypothalamus that you are no longer hungry—even a significant amount of time after you've ingested some protein. You can snort a line of chocolate chips and inhale all the potato chips you want, but neither one will make a dent in the hunger signals sent to your brain. Most women tend to crave and binge on carbs, but I've never had a client who binges on steak. Protein comes to the rescue, which offers our bodies a calming, sustained sense of satisfaction, and so our relationship to feeling hungry changes dramatically. Often when we crave starches at meals and sweets for dessert, we actually just need to increase our protein, quality fats, and fibers.

Getting an adequate amount of healthful protein daily also prompts your brain to produce the right mix of neurotransmitters to keep your mental focus razor-sharp. And starting your day with a protein-rich meal—two eggs and some turkey bacon—triggers the release of all sorts of happy chemicals, so you'll begin your workday feeling fit and energized.

Protein and Lean Muscle

You aren't going to get those taut, responsive muscles that you lust for if you don't eat enough protein, which provides the essential nutrients that allow the body to continuously fine-tune your cells and muscles. This, I know, seems to fly in the face of that old-time advice to load up on carbs in advance of a big workout or sporting event. Wrong. Eating protein—a vegetable omelet or a leftover steak—an hour before working out will give you the edge at the gym or on the playing field. Protein is your inner warrior goddess's best bet when it comes to being the lean, mean, fighting machine you yearn to be.

Splendor in the Grass

The principles for eating healthy proteins are the same as for produce: look for locally raised, ethically farmed, and organically nourished products. If you're going to become a cavewoman, then you're going to have to eat meat, fish, game, and eggs. Pastured cows (and sheep, and pigs, for that matter) provide the healthiest, most nutritious meat we can buy. Buffalo, elk, rabbit, ostrich, and bison also fit the bill. These animals get to roam around, take in the fresh air and sun, and feed on the native grasses and plants in the pastures.

Interestingly, grass-fed meat products tend to be lower in calories. According to *Pasture Perfect*, a book about grass-fed animals, a six-ounce cut of grass-fed beef can have 100 fewer calories (due to less fat) than the same cut from a grain-fed cow, contain higher levels of the very desirable omega-3 fatty acids, the antioxidants vitamins A and E, and up to seven times the amount of beta-carotene, a superpowerful antioxidant.

Free-Range Chic

I'm loving this trend of people raising chickens in their backyards. Chickens that are allowed to hunt and peck for their food on organic, untended plots of land get to indulge in a diet that's rich in grasses, bugs, worms, and other highly nutritious goodies. These birds tend to be leaner (usually having 20 percent less body fat), contain less saturated fat per pound, and contain a whopping 50 percent more vitamin A than their caged counterparts. The eggs of free-range, organic chickens also come superloaded for health, containing almost 35 percent less cholesterol, 10 percent less fat, 40 percent more vitamin A, and four times the omega-3 fatty acids than the standard USDA-approved egg.

Sustenance from the Sea

Eating fresh fish and shellfish is one of the healthiest things a Paleo girl can do. Fish, a food source bursting with lean protein, is rich in so many vital nutrients (bring on those omega-3 fatty acids!) that the Harvard School of Public Health has long recommended that we eat at least two servings of fresh fish per week. Why? Eating this baseline amount of fish can reduce a person's risk of developing heart disease by one-third. If you look at the data from across a wide array of studies, seafood consumption is credited with lowering the risk of death from heart disease by 36 percent. This is because the healthy oils found in fish such as salmon and mackerel seem to lubricate the blood in ways that reduce the likelihood of clotting, which can cause heart attacks and strokes. Researchers have estimated that ingesting the oils from these fish can reduce our overall risk of mortality by more than 15 percent.

The health benefits of eating fish aren't limited to the heart. Studies show that the omega-3 fatty acids, which are abundant in fish, provide our brains with the nutrients needed to ward off depression by prompting serotonin production. These fatty acids are also credited with keeping our skin and cells sleek and youthful and are also known to combat inflammation that may lead to joint pain and other ailments.

Go to the home-delivery company Vital Choice (www.vitalchoice.com) for wild-caught salmon and seafood that is remarkably clean and pristine. Trader Joe's and Whole Foods also offer wild Alaskan salmon; frozen at Trader's and fresh at Whole

Foods. If you can't buy fresh fish, purchase frozen fish to get the powerful nutritional benefits of seafood.

I can't stress enough how important it is to commit to eating a high-protein diet if you want to be as Paleo Chic as you can be. As with the other dietary changes I suggest throughout the book, give protein a chance—for at least a week or two—and you'll feel a remarkable shift in your energy and overall sense of well-being.

CHAPTER 7

The Skinny on Fat

I am a big believer in fat. I love chewing the fat with my girlfriends, and I definitely believe in the nutritional, healing value in healthy dietary fats. That's because I know how great good fats can make me look and feel.

I, too, was a longtime victim of the low-fat-food crazes that swept the land for so many years. In my late teens and early twenties, I literally starved myself of these healthful nutrients, and I found myself with wicked PMS and menstrual cramps. My skin had more spots than a leopard, and I toggled between Accutane and antibiotics to clear up the situation. If this way of eating was meant to make me healthier, I realized quickly that I was doomed.

Eating healthy saturated animal fats—those found in butter and lean, grass-fed meats, for example—is one of the best things you can do for your body. You don't even have to reach back to Paleo times for evidence of this. In the 1920s, Americans ate a high-fat diet loaded with meat, butter, and whole milk—and still had lower levels of coronary artery disease than we do now. Right around the time the Roaring Twenties gave way to the Great Depression, our kitchens became infiltrated by factory-produced, highly-processed foods. These "innovations" caused a raft of illnesses—including a bump in heart ailments. Since the 1950s, there has been a tremendous spike in the diagnoses of heart disease. All of a sudden, fat became the bad guy, and we lost sight of the healthy fats that our bodies need to function well.

Saturated fats help regulate our hormones, which you now know is at the heart of losing weight, building lean muscle mass, a glowing complexion, keeping our brains firing on all cylinders, protecting our vital organs, and making sure that our cells are replenished and toxin-free. It's time to wrestle to the ground the great American myth about dietary fat. Don't you ever wonder, *If fat-free is the way to go, why are we so fat?*

We can lose unwanted body fat only if we eat an adequate amount of healthful dietary fats. But how much is enough? You should be eating some dietary fat with every meal, which is why most of the recipes listed in this book have about 15 grams of fat (just over 1 tablespoon) per meal; this includes both the fat found within the protein source and the fat it's cooked in. And, you can also toss in another 10 grams per snack to allow for that ¼ cup of nuts or some coconut oil in your protein shake. Depending on your weight and body fat, you may need to go up or decrease accordingly, but I'm willing to bet that the starches you eat will have a far more detrimental impact on your body composition than the fats you are consuming.

It's important to learn the differences between good and bad fats so that you can eat the ones that are going to help you slim down. Here's what you need to know:

1. High-fat, high-protein, low-carb diets regulate blood sugar and insulin levels better than low-fat, high-carb diets can. Low-carb diets also raise levels of high-density lipoprotein (HDL, the "good" cholesterol), and decrease blood pressure.
2. Become knowledgeable about the fats you consume. Good fats are just that: good, not evil. Steer clear of trans fats, poor quality vegetable oils (see number 5 opposite),

hydrogenated oils, processed foods, and grain-fed meats. When you eat foods with high-quality fats, you can get 40 percent to 50 percent of your calories from fats and still lose weight. This may seem like a lot of calories from fat, but when you're not eating overprocessed, empty carbohydrates, your body needs another source of fuel in order to run optimally and stave off hunger.

3. Lowering body fat isn't only about your dietary fat intake. Whether or not you lose weight is also influenced by the quality of the proteins and carbs you eat. So make sure that you're eating grass-fed meats and organic eggs. Get the majority of your carbs from vegetables and fruits in the range of 100 grams per day. And say sayonara to sugar—as well as limit your intake of alcoholic beverages to one to two per week—if you want to lose weight.

4. Avoid all processed foods. Period.

5. Balance your omega-3 and omega-6 fats. Omega-3s are essential fatty acids found in fish and fish oil. Fish contain the omega-3s eicosapentaenoic acid (EPA), and docosahexaenoic acid (DHA). According to the National Research Council, more than sixty health conditions have been shown to benefit from fish oils. Omega-3s help reduce systemic and localized inflammation, treat dry skin, heart disease, depression, PMS, autoimmune conditions, and poor circulation, to name a few benefits.

It's important to have the right balance of different fats in your diet. Most sources of pro-inflammatory omega-6s can be found in vegetable, corn, cottonseed, safflower and sunflower oils, and should be avoided. However, there are a group of beneficial omega-6 fats, which are anti-inflammatory: black currant seed, borage, and evening primrose oil, found mostly in supplement form. The trick lies in keeping omega-6 fats in balance with omega-3s to the tune of at least a 3-to-1 ratio of omega-3 to omega-6 fats.

Most of us consume too many omega-6 fats and not enough omega-3 fats, due to our high consumption of vegetable oils coupled with eating grain-fed animals, corn, and soy; the typical American has a 20-to-1 ratio of omega-6s to omega-3s. This is a deal breaker for the human body!

Eggs from factory chickens contain twenty times more omega-6 fats than omega-3 fats, compared with organic, free-range chickens, which are rich in omega-3 fats. Farmed salmon contains more omega-6 fats than omega-3–rich wild Alaskan salmon do. Fish liver oil, fish eggs, egg yolks, organ meats, and seaweed are rich sources of omega-3s, but many people are unfamiliar with them, and so they don't cook or eat them.

Some people like to take flaxseed oil as an additional source of omega-3s. About 15 percent of the alpha linoleic acid in flaxseed oil will also convert to omega-3s in a healthy body. If you are diabetic, or your diet is too high in sugar, the conversion to EPA can be much more difficult. So relying on flax oil alone for omega-3 fatty acids can lead to a deficiency. It is also noteworthy that flax oil can raise men's levels of prostate-specific antigen (PSA), a biochemical marker used to screen for prostate cancer, so they should stick to ground flax for all of the benefits and none of the prostate problems.

Last but not least, let's also give a shout-out to an omega-6 fat called gamma linolenic acid. GLA has tremendous health-promoting effects and fights inflammation, skin conditions such as eczema and acne, and PMS. Evening primrose oil is another rich source of GLA. Taking GLA in conjunction with omega-3s will establish a healthy balance of essential fats from within.

Making Fat Work for You

Given the powerful regulatory benefits of fats, let's put them to work and keep you in skinny jeans! The following are my top ten favorite ways that fats will make you gorgeous from the inside out.

1. Healthy Fats Reduce PMS. Premenstrual syndrome is a condition of imbalances, often from inadequate amounts of omega-3s and other trace minerals found in fats that would otherwise help you feel calm and relaxed. Time for an oil change! Adding primrose oil and omega-3 fats, along with eating grass-fed meats and fish, can quench inflammatory fires from within and keep your hormones humming along smoothly. (Refer to the "Reproductive Hormone Balancing" protocol in chapter 11, page 184, for more information.)

2. Healthy Fats Balance Hormones. We require fat in our diets because fats are precursors to estrogen, progesterone, and testosterone. If we don't eat enough quality fats, we can feel depressed, experience changes in our menstrual cycle, get dry skin, and have a hard time burning our own body fat. We can also suffer from vaginal dryness and unnecessary menopausal symptoms. Insuring the proper balance of fats will keep your hormones in harmony.

3. Healthy Fats Fight Heart Disease. I explain this in greater detail on page 90, but suffice it to say that there is no conclusive relationship between saturated fat intake and coronary artery disease. The message has been botched for years; we need to return to our roots on this one.

4. Healthy Fats Regulate Inflammation. When you remove quality oils from food and replace them with poor-quality oils such as canola or corn, you ignite your inner inflammatory fires. Margarine and trans fats literally block healthy fats from being absorbed by our bodies! If you have junk fats in your diet, it can take up to two years to displace those bad fats with healthy ones at the cellular level. There is no time like the present for getting those toxic fats out of your system and replacing them with healthy ones.

5. Healthy Fats Are Necessary for Fat Loss. When you remove natural fats from foods and replace them with sugar, you can become insulin resistant. On the other hand, if you eat enough of the right kinds of fats, you can improve your insulin sensitivity and stoke your metabolic fire. Omega-3s help ignite the genes that burn fat and turn off the genes that store fat. Plus, the medium-chain triglycerides found in coconut oil (a champion fat) help the body naturally burn fat more efficiently.

6. Healthy Fats Control Hunger and Cravings. Eliminating fat and cholesterol starves the body of nutrients it needs and messes with the hunger-fullness messages it sends to the brain. When your body is deprived of fat, your brain tells it to go into famine mode, damaging your metabolism and converting every calorie it can latch onto into stored fat. As your brain biochemistry goes wonky, serotonin levels drop, and your cravings pick up speed so fast that you'll be sucking down that chocolate milkshake before you know it.

7. Healthy Fats Promote Bone Density. We know we need calcium for healthy, strong bones. We also need saturated fats to transport that calcium to our bones, which is why raw, full-fat dairy products (see page 113) are a much better option for those who can tolerate dairy. Without saturated fat to transport it, all the calcium you get from dark leafy greens won't do you much good.

8. Healthy Fats Give You Glowing Skin. Dry skin isn't a lotion deficiency—it's an essential fatty acid deficiency! To get to the root of the problem, you need to lube up from the inside out: a combination of 2,000 milligrams primrose oil and 3,000 milligrams omega-3 fats will help. The cool thing is that if you're at the opposite end of the spectrum and have oily skin, this combo of omega-3s and primrose oil will also control sebum production and level out your skin's oil production.

9. Healthy Fats Support Thyroid Function. Omega-3 fatty acids help improve thyroid hormone signaling pathways in the liver, which means that the precious thyroid hormones in our bodies will reach their targeted cells. Omega-3s also help ease inflammation that is secondary to thyroid dysfunction. Cooking with coconut oil also has the potential to greatly improve thyroid system function because it stimulates the metabolism and boosts energy.

10. Healthy Fats Relieve Depression. Brain tissue is composed of 60 percent fat, so feeding the correct fats to the brain on a daily basis boosts serotonin naturally. Omega-3s also fight inflammation in the gut, which is the primary place of serotonin and other neurotransmitter production. Treating the gut and the brain simultaneously can help nip depression in the bud.

Saturate Yourself in Healthy Fats

In the Paleolithic era, our ancestors ate saturated fats because they were available in meats critical to their vitality. Today the public runs screaming from them, fearing that they'll kill us. (When was the last time a doctor encouraged you to have more butter? I thought so.) Saturated fats stay solid at room temperature and can be found in all sorts of delicious places, such as marbled cuts of meat, butter, and coconut oil. And contrary to popular belief, which is not based on any science, there is *no* conclusive evidence that saturated fat increases the risk of heart disease—especially if you eat fat from grass-fed animals.

The real head-scratcher in all of this is that plasma-saturated fat (saturated fat found in the blood)—the presumed cause for our concern with fat—is actually a product of the *carbohydrates* you take in, not the dietary saturated fats you eat. The polyunsaturated fats that are found in isolated oils such as corn, vegetable, cottonseed, canola, soybean, safflower, and sunflower are not—I repeat, are not—healthy saturated fats; they are disruptive to our bodies.

Today we get 20 percent or more of our calories from polyunsaturated fatty acids, which gum up the metabolism when they replace quality fats in our cell membranes. The problem with poly-unsaturated fats is that they're extremely fragile and lack the chemical stability of saturated fats, so when we remove them from their whole-food sources and use them as isolated oils, they produce free radicals in the body. And when they're used in cooking, they break down further and become even more loaded with free radicals. Saturated fats—the safest oils for cooking—don't harm us in this way. Saturated fats are stable at room temperature and when heated. In fact, coconut oil kept at room temperature for a year will show no signs of rancidity or degradation at all.

Saturated fats are necessary for optimal health. They comprise at least 50 percent of cell membranes and contain huge amounts of the essential fat-soluble vitamins A, D, E, and K. They protect the liver from toxins, enhance immunity, are necessary for proper function of the kidneys and lungs, and help us utilize essential fatty acids. The short-chain saturated fatty acids (found in butter and coconut oil) are antimicrobial—they help fight against bacteria, yeast, and parasites and support the immune system. Some cultures selectively hunted animals with the most fat, because animal fat was highly prized for its medicinal benefits.

Aside from being good for you, saturated fat is also good for your workouts, where it can be used for immediate energy. We've unlearned the art of trusting our bodies where fat is concerned, and as a result, we've missed out on saturated fat as a fantastic source of energy. In fact, excess carbohydrates get stored as *saturated body fat*, so all of the so-called experts pointing fingers at saturated fat as dangerous are misguided. Saturated fats do not increase tri-glycerides; carbohydrates do. The ratio of HDL to triglycerides and the size of our cholesterol particles are far more predictive of cardiovascular disease. We must take a look at the real culprits of heart disease and stop vilifying natural, whole foods we've been eating for millions of years and should still be eating today.

I have not found any credible peer-reviewed, controlled studies that link saturated fat intake to cancer; only questionnaires asking cancer patients what they have eaten over the past five years can shed any light at all on this presumed connection. The studies suggest that a diet high in unsaturated fats, processed grains, sugar, margarine, vegetable oils, starches, and grain-fed meats aren't good for us. Comprehensive breast cancer studies also show no correlation between eating a low-fat diet and a reduced risk of breast cancer.

If you were going to a red carpet event, you wouldn't buy just any old frock off the rack; you'd want to look and feel your best in a designer gown, right? Well, think of saturated fats as the ultimate couture dress for your body; they will keep your body gorgeously balanced and healthy from the inside out. From the beginning of our lives, we drink mother's milk, which contains 54 percent saturated fat and is essential for brain development. Our hearts naturally prefer to be fed saturated fats instead of carbohydrates for energy. Our bones need saturated fats to assimilate calcium properly. Our hormone production is dictated by our saturated fat intake. Saturated fats also help to enhance the body's defense against disease. Viruses and fungi such as candida don't stand a chance with the presence of lauric acid in coconut oil and myristic acid in butter! Our livers need saturated fats to protect against toxins, medications, and booze. Our lungs need saturated fats to prevent asthma and other breathing disorders. Our bodies need saturated fats to feel fuller and stay lean. Greater satiety means that you'll eat fewer carbohydrates and less junk and poor-quality fats.

Fats That Paleo Chic Girls Love

I hope you love your fat—even if you want to shed it. But that's not the fat I'm talking about. We Paleo girls love, love, love our healthy dietary fats. They make us the lean, mean fighting machines we need to be to rock our incredibly rich and vibrant lives. Here are my all-time favorite Paleo Chic fats:

Avocado
Beef tallow and fat (found on grass-fed meats)
Butter (from the milk of grass-fed cows)
Chia seeds
Chicken fat
Coconut (raw) and coconut oil (see sidebar)
Duck and goose fat
Flaxseeds (ground)
Grapeseed Oil
Lard
Olives and olive oil
Nuts and seeds (raw and butters, especially sunflower,
    pumpkin, and sesame seeds, almonds, walnuts, pistachios,
    hazelnuts, Brazil nuts, pecans, cashews, and macadamia
    nuts)
Sesame oil (toasted)

NUTS FOR COCONUTS

Coconut oil is the most perfect fat that a girl can possibly consume. Once vilified, coconut oil is a stable and nutritious fat.

- It's surprisingly rich in short-chain and medium-chain fatty acids, which make it a natural fat-loss nutrient for the body. It reduces the stress from oxidative damage to cells, which makes it the perfect preworkout food.

- Through its antiviral properties, coconut oil boosts immune function and lowers the body's histamine, or inflammatory trigger, response. It bypasses the gut and goes right to the liver for absorption. Because the body uses it immediately, the oil can even be given to people on tube feedings. Coconut oil also slows down the aging of the skin from the inside out. Both eating and using it as a moisturizer will do your body good!

- In the early 1940s, farmers used inexpensive coconut oil for fattening their animals, but they found that it made the livestock lean, active, and hungry fat-burning machines instead. By the late 1940s, it was discovered that feeding animals soybeans and corn made them fatter, and they ate less food. So began one of the great causes of inflammation and obesity in this country.

- Eating coconut oil regularly and cutting down on starchy foods can naturally lower your cholesterol. Doing so lowers cholesterol by promoting its conversion into pregnenolone—the grand precursor hormone from which almost all of the other steroid hormones are made—including DHEA, progesterone, testosterone, estrogen, and cortisol. Coconut-eating cultures have consistently lower cholesterol numbers than Americans do.

- You can purchase organic coconut oil in supermarkets, health food stores, and chains such as Trader Joe's and Whole Foods Market. It will become solid at cooler temperatures and either softer or completely liquid at warmer temperatures. You can use it for sautéing, baking, or in your postworkout smoothie. Store it in a cool, dark place for optimal freshness; it will easily keep for up to one year—no refrigeration required.

I want you to march to the grocery store and buy these fats. Purge your pantry of these bad fats: canola, corn, vegetable, sunflower, safflower, soybean, peanut and/or cottonseed oils. (Phew!) Anything fried. All margarines or butter-substitute spreads. Partially hydrogenated oils. Vegetable shortenings. There—don't you feel lighter already?

Now that you're back on track with fat, it's time for us to get down to the nitty-gritty: the Paleo Chic diet. When you turn the page, there will be no turning back, and you'll be on your way to rocking a seriously healthy, seriously hot body before you know it.

PART 3

Cavewomen Don't Get Fat

CHAPTER 8

The Paleo Detox

Camp Detox: The First Fourteen Days

Although *detox* is a hot buzzword these days, it's something that you need to do on a daily basis to lighten your body's toxic load. During the two-week Paleo Detox, you will take a step back from carbohydrates to resensitize your body to insulin and rebalance your hunger-fullness hormones. This will also give your brain the chance to change the way you think about food, and your body the chance to adjust to your new way of eating. Lastly, the Paleo Detox will also give your body time to deplete some of your glycogen stores from muscle tissue and ultimately make your cheat day more effective. (See chapter 9 for more info on the cheat meal.)

Staying within the Paleo Detox parameters for the first two weeks of the entire plan is key. You can come back to this phase at different times throughout the year. Also, use—and stick to—this program two weeks before a big event, like a wedding or a college reunion, to make sure that sexy dress you bought still fits.

During these two weeks, you can lose five to eight pounds of puffiness and bloating. Your body will start releasing toxins stored in fat cells and shed excess water weight while building lean mus-

cle mass. This phase also gives your gut a break from most allergenic foods and quenches your body with antioxidants and trace
minerals.

K.I.S.S. (Keep It Simple, Sister!)

Do you know that many people find that it's easier to do their
taxes than figure out what to eat? Food companies have done such
a successful job at sending us confusing messages that no one
knows what to put in her mouth anymore. Most people believe
that a low-fat muffin is healthier than two eggs fried in butter,
even though the muffin is made with 100 percent processed ingredients, while the eggs are completely natural. Knowing what
foods to eat has become way too complicated! So I'm going to
make it easy for you. I've researched every ingredient and nutritional recommendation in this book and made sure they contain
no processed foods.

THE PALEO GIRL FOOD MANIFESTO

1. Eat Only Real Foods. Annemarie Colbin, the founder and CEO
who runs the culinary school the Natural Gourmet Institute, in
New York City, says, "If it doesn't run, fly, swim, or grow from the
ground, it's not food!" Kudos, Annemarie, I'm right there with you.
We need to eat foods that are in their original state. Once we start
mucking up our foods with processed gunk, they are no longer
nutritious or real.

If you read a food label with fifteen ingredients, and you can't
even pronounce half of them, put it back on the shelf. If a packaged food has more than five ingredients, don't buy it. And if the
food packaging or the ingredients inside are in colors not found in
nature, you can bet that a major food conglomerate manufactures
it. If it's produced by a major food conglomerate, you need to be

particularly careful that it contains only ingredients that help your cause in feeling good or getting lean.

2. Restock Your Produce Often. Fresh foods are just that: fresh. Hunter-gatherers had no storage facilities, so they immediately ate what they caught and killed or picked from trees and bushes. We now have the luxury to buy many kinds of foods and cook, refrigerate and freeze, and reheat them. At farmers' markets, we can purchase foods that were picked that morning, as compared to grocery store produce that was picked ten days prior and warehoused until put on the shelves. Wherever you buy your produce, eat it as quickly as possible to obtain its best nutritional value. Fresh food spoils quickly, so plan your week of eating accordingly. If you find that your produce is reaching the end of its shelf life and you just can't get to preparing it in time, freeze what you can or cook it and then freeze it. Wasting food and hard-earned money would be a shame. If you have time, consider smaller and more frequent trips to the produce aisle for the freshest options available.

When it comes to meat, I suggest ordering it online at Eatwild (www.eatwild.com)—a comprehensive resource for humanely raised wild game, beef, eggs, and raw milk—or making a monthly visit to your butcher and stocking up. If you have the space for an industrial or chest freezer, look into buying and sharing a whole or half of a cow, lamb, or pig with friends or buying a portion from a local farm that raises grass-fed animals. The meat can be butchered into various cuts, wrapped, and labeled to keep in the freezer for six months. Thaw meat over several days in the refrigerator before cooking.

3. Prepare Your Food in Batches. I love to cook for my family, but not every night! I double or triple recipes when I make meat sauces or soups so that I can serve or use them throughout the week in different ways. Or I make large batches of stews and braises, and then freeze the leftovers in containers and use them as needed. A cook's tip: if you chill containers of food in the fridge before freezing them, you'll avoid accumulating those dreaded ice crystals and subsequent freezer burn.

4. Get the Veg Edge. Jeannette Bessinger, clean food coach and creator of the recipes in *The Healthiest Meals on Earth: The Surprising, Unbiased Truth About What Meals to Eat and Why*, taught me that vegetables are essential for variety when it comes to low-carb eating. Plus, eating lots of vegetables fills you up, and they are great sources of fiber and water. Vegetables also provide a wide range of flavors—sweet, salty, sour, bitter, and pungent—to help reduce postmeal cravings. And while your jaws are working overtime to chew up fibrous greens, the eating process naturally slows down, so you can taste what you're eating and allow your body to begin predigesting your food. Aim for 6 cups of raw vegetables and 2 cups cooked per day.

5. Purchase the Best Quality Food You Can Afford. If health is a priority in your life, your grocery bill can wind up on the high side. There are plenty of ways to make good food affordable. Buy in bulk. Buy locally. Join a CSA (community-supported agriculture) to support local farmers. Cooking your food, rather than buying precooked meals, will save you tons of money. Do your best to buy grass-fed meats and organic produce; they are the cheapest health insurance plan you'll ever purchase!

6. Know the Codes. Ever wonder what those strings of numbers mean that you find on stickers on fresh produce? These PLU ("price lookup") codes enable farmers and produce companies to store information about the fresh produce that we consume.

A four-digit code beginning with a 3 or a 4 indicates that the produce is "conventionally grown." This could indicate the use or presence of agricultural fertilizers, industrial chemicals and/or pesticides during production. A five-digit code beginning with a 9 means the product was grown organically. To be certified as organic produce, the product must comply with specific standards, such as the absence of synthetic pesticides and chemical fertilizers. A five-digit code starting with the number 8 means that the produce is "genetically modified"—also known as "GM foods" "biotech foods" or "Frankenfoods."

7. Practice Mind-Full Eating. Eating is one of the most intricate acts we perform as humans. Eating is emotionally and physiologically driven, and how and what we eat are direct reflections of who we are and how we think about food. If we shove food into our mouths while watching TV or arguing with our kids, then we're not allowing our food to do what it should: nourish and sustain us. If, however, we allow ourselves to think about how a certain food will make us feel after we eat it, we're likely to make better choices and take better care of ourselves. Mindful eating is about sitting down at the table without distractions—no TV, no smart phones—and focusing on the food in front of you. It means eating slowly and savoring each bite that someone took the time to prepare. For me, eating is also about gratitude. Whenever I sit down to a meal, I thank my lucky stars that I am able to enjoy such healthful food and take great care of my body. Dr. Deanna Minich, author of *The Complete Handbook of Quantum Healing: An A–Z Self-Healing Guide for over 100 Common Ailments*, taught me to set the tone for meals by saying a positive word before eating, such as *gratitude, love,* or *peace,* since pleasure can help us absorb the nutrients from our food. Now that's what I call nutrition for the soul!

8. Listen to Your Body. Eat when you are hungry and stop when you are full. I advocate eating five times a day to keep blood sugar level and fend off cravings. This kind of preemptive eating keeps our blood sugar and moods gloriously stable, preventing you from becoming ravenous and inhaling everything in sight. But if you just can't do that—some people say that eating the Paleo way allows more food than they want to eat—that's okay too. You know your body better than I do. While eating protein-rich foods is important, it's even more important to know your own comfort zone. If 6 ounces of protein is too much, but 4 ounces seems right, then go with that. Bear in mind that your appetite will rise and fall throughout the month along with your estrogen levels. Be sure to trust your body on the days you feel hungrier. It all evens out in the end!

9. Enjoy a Cheat Meal Once Per Week. A cheat meal, which allows you to eat anything you want, is a great way to boost your metabolism and your leptin levels, and ultimately regulate hunger and body fat levels. Diets, especially low-calorie ones, tend to lower leptin levels. This causes extreme hunger and tells your body to hang on for dear life to fat, thinking it needs that unnecessary fat to survive in the future. Since leptin levels are directly linked to caloric intake, spiking up those calories during a cheat meal will mix things up and keep your body guessing. If your body understands that you're increasing your calorie intake and food is plentiful, it will let go of fat effortlessly. Be judicious here, because sometimes a cheat meal can trigger cravings for a few days afterward. I personally find that drinking a couple glasses of wine is much easier for me to bounce back from than eating a slice of bread or cake. Over time, you'll discover exactly what works for you.

YOUR FOOD JOURNAL

The best way to get a handle on your eating is to keep a food journal. I recommend keeping a hunger-fullness log to check in before, during, and after a meal. At the beginning of each meal, track your hunger and fullness on a scale of 1 to 10, where 1 is famished and 10 is stuffed. You want to ideally start eating at a 3 and stop at a 6. Practice eating every three hours and keeping track of where you fall on the spectrum; you never want to let yourself get too hungry or too full. Record yourself before eating, midmeal, and again at the end of the meal.

Also, it's important to develop habits that signal your meal is over. Pop a breath mint, brush your teeth, have a cup of herbal tea, or anything else that signals it's time to move on.

Ready, Set, Go!

Next, I want you to take a close look at what's in your pantry and fridge and clean it out. Removing any roadblocks in the form of processed foods means that decision making will be oh-so-much easier when it comes to putting together your meals. If there are no crackers in your kitchen, then you won't be tempted to eat them. Ditto for all flour-based foods: cookies, snack foods, candy, cereals, pasta, muffins, bread, white rice, and processed grains. Get rid of them. They get in your way by raising your circulating insulin level and disrupting the hormonal balance that helps your body shed fat.

If family members or roommates don't want to join you in the Paleo Chic diet, keep your food in a separate cupboard. Stock your pantry with jerky, spices, nuts, nut butters, salsa, and organic canned tomatoes, olives, artichoke hearts, and coconut oil. Fill your fridge with all types of fresh produce, fats, and proteins. Here's the list of everything you'll need to get started:

SHOPPING LIST

Proteins (Grass-Fed Meats, Poultry, and Eggs Are Best)

Beef	Bison
Beef, bison, venison, elk jerky (grass fed)	Chicken
	Duck

Eggs
Elk
Fatty cold-water fish:
    sardines, mackerel,
    herring, cod
Lamb
Nitrate- and gluten-free deli
    meat (Applegate Farms)
Pork
Rabbit

Sausages (no fillers,
    gluten-free)
Shellfish (escargots, shrimps,
    oysters, mussels, lobster,
    clams)
Turkey
Venison
Wild Alaskan salmon (filet,
    canned, smoked)

DIY JERKY

Making your own jerky is a snap. It's delish, nutrish, and plain ol' fun! These ain't your momma's Slim Jims—these are the real deal. So grab a hunk of meat, flip on your oven, and let's get cracking!

Choose a lean cut of grass-fed meat such as flank steak or London broil, since cuts with more fat means that the meat can quickly turn rancid. Ask your butcher to cut 1 pound of meat into ¼-inch strips against the grain.

Preheat oven to 150°F or as low as yours will go. Heat 2 tablespoons coconut aminos, 1 crushed garlic clove, 1 tablespoon raw honey, and 1 teaspoon onion powder in a saucepan. Bring to a boil, reduce heat, and add the meat strips. Simmer for 2 minutes. Remove the meat from the saucepan and dry with paper towels.

Arrange the meat strips on a wire rack set on a baking sheet.

Bake 6 to 8 hours, turning once halfway through. The jerky is done when it turns dark and cracks when it is bent.

Cool and store jerky in clean jars, or wrap it in freezer paper and freeze it. Will keep for two to three months.

Carbohydrates
Vegetables

Arugula
Asparagus
Beets
Broccoli
Broccoli rabe
Brussels sprouts
Cabbage
Carrots
Cauliflower
Celery
Collard greens
Cucumbers
Eggplant
Endive
Garlic
Green beans

Kale
Leeks
Lettuces (arugula, Boston,
    butter, radicchio, romaine)
Mushrooms
Onions
Pepper
Radishes
Shallots
Snap peas
Spinach
Sprouts (bean sprouts,
    broccoli sprouts)
Tomatoes
Zucchini

Starchy Vegetables (These Count as Carbohydrates)

Acorn squash
Butternut squash
Parsnips
Plantains

Spaghetti squash
Sweet potato (yam)
Taro
Turnips

Fresh Fruits

Apples
Apricots
Berries
Cantaloupes
Cherries
Clementines
Grapefruits

Kiwis
Lemons
Limes
Oranges
Peaches
Pears
Plums

You Can Eat One of These Fruits Once a Day, Preferably Post Workout

Banana	Papaya
Grapes	Pineapple
Mango	Watermelon

Fats

Nuts and seeds: Raw almonds, Brazil nuts, cashews, hazelnuts, macadamia nuts, pecans, pine nuts, pistachios, walnuts, chia seeds, flaxseeds, pumpkin seeds, sesame seeds, sunflower seeds. (Store in airtight containers in the freezer to prevent them from turning rancid.)

Nut and seed butters: especially sunflower, pumpkin, and sesame seeds, almonds, walnuts, pistachios, hazelnuts, Brazil nuts, pecans, cashews, and macadamia nuts—all of which are rich in trace minerals and quality fats.

Almond meal	Unsalted butter and clarified
Avocado	butter from grass-fed
Coconut flakes (unsweetened)	cows (Kerrygold brand)
Coconut oil	Heavy cream from grass-fed
Chicken fat	cows
Duck fat	Lard
Olives	Chicken fat (schmaltz)
Extra-virgin olive oil	Beef tallow
Grapeseed oil	

Condiments

Organic beef, chicken, and	Dried spices (gluten- and
vegetable broths	soy-free)
Mustard	Organic tomato paste
Hot sauce	Extra-virgin olive oil
Horseradish	Vinegar (balsamic, apple cider,
Fresh herbs	white)
Coconut aminos	Wasabi

Hydration
Water! Water! Water!

Green and black teas

Organic coffee

Hot cocoa made from water,
  unsweetened cocoa

powder, and stevia

Seltzer

Almond and coconut milk
  (unsweetened)

Coconut water (unsweetened)

Baking Ingredients
Almond flour

Butter

Cocoa powder

Coconut flour

Coconut oil

Grapeseed oil

Honey

Pecan flour

Stevia

Xylitol

CHANGE TAKES PRACTICE

After so many years as a practicing nutritionist who follows her own advice, I forget sometimes how hard it can be to change your eating habits. When I advise clients to clear out gluten, I usually hear two different responses when I review their food diaries. Client A will say to me, "Everywhere I look, I see limitations." Client B will say to me, "Everywhere I look, I see options."

How can two people see the world of eating from such different ends of the spectrum? I call it selective editing. Simply defined, we prioritize the work we are ready to do and draw a line in the sand for what we won't. We are our own rate-limiting reactions; although we often stand in our own way, we can also learn to clear a path to our successes.

Change can be hard—especially if you're not ready for it. When you live on Pirate's Booty cheese puff snacks, it can rock your world when you start eating nuts, steak, and spinach instead. Becoming a hunter-gatherer takes fortitude and practice, and for most people, it's a very gradual process. Fortunately, our minds are programmable homing devices for tracking Paleo-style foods. We may not be wired for immediate change, but we are certainly capable of gradually embracing a new lifestyle.

We are either victimized by our choices or empowered by them. So if you feel like you're following someone else's plan, then your choices will never feel like a lifestyle for you. Telling yourself, "My nutritionist told me I can't eat this," versus "I'm going to choose foods that help me get lean," have two very different messages. If you are ready to embrace change, and it actually feels like a choice for you, then the world is your oyster—and quite a delicious one at that!

BFFFs (Best Friends Forever Foods)

Protein and fiber-rich vegetables are your BFFFs (Best Friends Forever Foods) when it comes to preserving lean muscle mass. Without adequate protein intake, you'll lose muscle mass, which can lead to systemic inflammation and a surge of stress hormones, as well as a slower metabolism and an increase in body fat. Eating dietary protein preserves metabolically active muscle mass while keeping your brain biochemistry in check. That means you'll feel great through better body composition, sleep, moods, and hormonal balance.

As I mentioned in chapter 6, you should aim for at least 1 ounce of protein per pound of body weight. So if you weigh 150 pounds, eat 150 grams of protein per day. There are 7 grams of protein in an ounce, so 150 grams of protein equals 21 ounces per day. This means that you can eat an average of 5 ounces at meals, and another 2 to 3 ounces for each snack.

If you're worried you're going to be increasing your calories and gaining weight, don't be. The Paleo Chic plan is all about hormonal balance, which ultimately retrains your body to burn calories efficiently while burning body fat. Rest assured you will not be dramatically increasing your calories, but you can still reduce your body fat, have greater endurance during your workouts, and feel fuller for longer amounts of time. Which means fewer cravings and less dependence on stimulants just to get you through the day. Remember, your diet will dictate 80 percent of your body changes and help you build lean muscle; exercise helps you stay lean and drives insulin into cells for the remaining 20 percent of fat loss.

Greens Goddess

Greens are an essential part of the Paleo diet. Nutritious greens— dark, leafy ones such as kale, spinach, arugula, and others—clean up your liver, quench any inflammatory fires in your intestinal tract, give you gorgeous skin, and tons of energy.

What can greens do for you?

- Detoxify environmental estrogens and help prevent cancer.
- Provide a boost of antioxidants and stimulate enzymes that detoxify the body.
- Render harmful substances such as booze and tobacco into waste products that the body can eliminate.
- Protect against environmental carcinogens by binding to toxins and deactivating them.
- Stimulate digestion, regulate appetite and sugar cravings, and promote weight loss.

Liquid Green

Most of us don't eat enough greens on a daily basis, so green juices are a quick and easy way to get a healthy dose of their nutrients. But use them to *supplement* your vegetable intake; there's no replacement for fresh, fibrous, green vegetables!

I recommend you drink green juices three times per day for the first two weeks of your Paleo Detox.

There are three ways you can drink your greens:

1. freshly juiced in a juicer;
2. blended together in a Vitamix blender, which combines whole vegetables and leaves the fiber intact; and
3. powdered greens added to a glass of water or to a postworkout smoothie.

No matter what your choice, your body will thank you with renewed energy, a trimmer waistline, digestive wellness, and glowing skin.

"But Esther," you ask, "the thought of drinking greens daily makes me want to hurl! Can't I just eat a lot of vegetables every day instead?" I never ask my clients and readers to do anything that I wouldn't do myself. So hear me out on this one, because it's easier and more pleasant than you think. The reality is that in the world we live in, we all need to drink our greens on a daily basis to keep our bodies running smoothly and detoxify all the chemicals we're exposed to daily. And volumewise, a tall glass of juice can expose your body to three times the amount of vegetables that go into a juice than you can ever fit inside your stomach or actually have time to eat. So jump in, kids, and let's get those feet wet! Here is my favorite straight-up, no-nonsense green drink that will leave you fresh as a daisy and energized for the day:

THE GREEN GANGSTA

Serves one

1 cup spinach   1 cucumber
2 cups kale   1 celery stalk
2 cups parsley

Put all ingredients in juicer or Vitamix; add 1 cup water if you are using a Vitamix.

Drink immediately.

If using powdered greens, purchase one flavored naturally with mint or lemon-lime. I recommend PaleoGreens by Designs for Health. Each tablespoon of powder provides a hefty dose of organic greens that have been processed at a low temperature to keep all the active enzymes intact. I take some with me when I travel and dump some into my postworkout shake if I don't have any fresh greens on hand.

Smooth Moves with Fiber

Think fiber isn't glamorous or sexy? You might change your mind once you have a flat stomach and gain control over your hunger and your cravings. Getting enough fiber will keep your digestive system humming along smoothly with regular bowel movements and less gas and bloating. Fiber helps build the "good" bacteria, or probiotics, in your system, which, in turn, helps your body make digestive enzymes. Fiber also bulks up your bowel movements and enables them to pass through more quickly.

One of the most common reasons that women come to see me is constipation. As we do some detective work into their digestive history, often these women have a history of antibiotic use and have either been on or still take oral contraceptives. What does either medication have to do with your digestion? Everything. When you take antibiotics, you wipe out the offending bacteria that are causing problems, but you also wipe the good bacteria from your intestines as well. The pill can also cause a bacterial imbalance in the intestinal tract, allowing yeast overgrowth. Fiber to the rescue! It is crucial in restoring digestive balance and enables healthy bacteria to recolonize the gut.

Fiber is also a crucial component of hormonal balance. It binds to estrogen in the intestinal tract so that the body can excrete it. The lignans in flaxseeds are phytoestrogens (estrogen-like plant compounds) that can act like estrogen at low doses but block estrogen at higher doses. So if you're suffering from wicked PMS each month or are heading down the menopause highway, incorporate some ground flax and chia seeds into your diet to reduce your circulating estrogen levels.

How much fiber should you aim for daily? As much as you can tolerate, but eat at least 30 grams per day. Excellent high-fiber choices are 2 tablespoons of freshly ground flax or chia seeds (4 and 7 grams of fiber, respectively), dark green leafy vegetables, sweet potatoes and winter squash, and fresh fruits. The average American eats only 12 grams of fiber per day and just isn't eating enough of rough stuff. So make sure you're eating at least 6 to 8 cups raw vegetables per day, or 3 to 4 cups cooked. And if that's just too much food to put in your stomach, or you don't have the time to get it down your gullet, toss some of those veggies into a Vitamix and drink up.

Where Do These Foods Fit in with Paleo Plans?

While it's true that cavewomen did not have access to agricultural foods, we modern women do, which can make for some grey areas within the Paleo plans. So if you tolerate the foods listed below, you can incorporate them into your eating plans. If not, you should avoid them altogether or enjoy them as an occasional indulgence. I am not putting a Paleo stamp of approval on these foods, mind you, but I am making an exception because I recognize that these foods can exist within a dietary loophole of Paleo eating. Ultimately, the Paleo lifestyle needs to be sustainable, and that may mean that some loopholes exist.

Dairy

Back in the good ol' Paleo days, the only milk our ancestors drank was breast milk until they were weaned. In contemporary times, however, milk, cheese, yogurt, and other dairy products are part of many diets. Lactase is an enzyme that helps break down lactose, another enzyme that makes it possible to digest milk. While some Europeans have no trouble producing lactase, almost every other ethnic group stops producing lactase at an early age. For this reason, cow's milk and other dairy products cause digestive problems in people with lactose intolerance. (Some people can tolerate goat's or sheep's milk.) When they do eat them, they often become nauseous, bloated, or develop diarrhea. Even if you do tolerate milk, proceed with caution: many studies have linked consumption of pasteurized milk with exacerbation of lactose intolerance, allergies, asthma, frequent ear infections, gastrointestinal problems, diabetes, autoimmune disease, attention deficit/hyperactivity disorder, and constipation. Just one glass of commercial milk can contain a cocktail of up to twenty painkillers, antibiotics, and growth hormones, not to mention omega-6 fats and residues of GMO corn and soy fed to the cows. No, thank you!

We also have to take into account the hormonal effects of milk and dairy products. Because milk is rich in carbs (12 grams per 8 ounces), it will raise your insulin level after you drink it—especially if it's low fat or fat-free. Many athletes use milk in their postworkout shake for this very reason. But if you're not very active, and you drink at least three to four glasses of milk per day, that's an automatic recipe for weight gain and fat storage.

MILK

Raw milk is easier to digest than pasteurized milk because it is rich in probiotics and maintains the balance of healthy bacteria in the gut. In addition, raw milk contains phosphatase enzymes, which help the body absorb calcium. Raw milk from grass-fed cows will also help keep you lean, since it is rich in the powerful antioxidant conjugated linoleic acid (CLA) and omega-3s, which naturally help the body burn fat. And raw milk contains protein, trace minerals, and every known fat and water-soluble vitamin. (To find raw milk near you, go to the website A Campaign for Real Milk (www.real-milk.com.) This website is the work of the Weston A. Price Foundation, a nutrition education foundation that supports the research of Dr. Weston A. Price and a diet rich in whole foods and saturated animal fats.

Once milk is pasteurized, it's a whole different story. The beneficial bacteria are destroyed, the calcium can no longer be absorbed, and the raw enzymes become denatured. If you can't tolerate milk products, ask yourself if it's the type of animal whose milk you are consuming or the pasteurization process.

We now know that grass-fed cows produce quality dairy products. Aside from the heart-healthy saturated fats present, quality dairy foods are chock-full of the bone-building vitamin K2, omega-3 fatty acids, and as you now know, CLA. I'm not telling you to consume sticks of butter, mind you, but should you decide to consume dairy, make sure that it's the best you can find.

CHEESE

The best cheeses for you are goat cheese, feta cheese, sheep's-milk cheese, buffalo-milk cheese, and any raw, unpasteurized cheeses you can find; goat, sheep, and buffalo-milk cheese are usually better tolerated by people who have allergies or sensitivities to cow's milk. And unpasteurized cheeses are richer in calcium than the more processed brands, since the pasteurization process makes it difficult for calcium to be absorbed by the body.

YOGURT

Yogurt is a fermented form of dairy rich in probiotics, which are live microorganisms present in our intestinal tracts that facilitate digestion, keep our immune system healthy, synthesize nutrients, and support the development and functioning of the gut. Fermented dairy is one of the best forms of dairy to eat or drink, because most of the sugars present get consumed during the fermentation process. Healthy people normally have about four pounds of beneficial bacteria in their intestinal tracts, and yogurt helps keep that balance intact. Yogurt is low in lactose and easy to digest. So if you eat yogurt, make sure that it's the full-fat variety from the milk of either a goat, sheep, or cow; fat-free dairy products register as carbs in the body and raise insulin levels. And skip the sugary varieties with fruit; add some fresh berries, slivered almonds, and stevia if you need a sweet fix.

BUTTER AND HEAVY CREAM

Butter and heavy cream are some of my favorite fats. And although they fall within the dairy family, they are comprised mostly of saturated fat, with just a trace of lactose. So putting a splash of heavy cream in your coffee or cooking your vegetables in butter doesn't pose a problem for most people. But let's say that you want to up your clean game one step further. This would be an opportune time to get to know ghee, a butter that has been clarified. This means that all milk solids have been removed, and what's left is pure, delicious, and healthy butterfat. It stands up better to high-heat cooking than butter, and will keep fresh for long periods of time. So unless you are managing autoimmune conditions or severe food allergies, enjoy butter and heavy cream from grass-fed cows, or keep it squeaky clean with ghee.

To make your own ghee, place unsalted butter in a saucepan over medium heat until it becomes foamy. Once the foam settles, there will be white specks in the butter that soon turn brown. Put the bottom of the saucepan in cold water. Strain the butter through a coffee filter or double piece of cheesecloth into a measuring cup or a small dish. The clear—clarified—butter will drip to the bottom. Discard the coffee filter with the milk solids. Use the clarified butter immediately or cover and refrigerate until needed.

To make 100 percent dairy-free whipped cream, use coconut cream instead of heavy cream. Open a can of full-fat coconut milk and scoop out the thick cream at the top and put it in a bowl. Add ½ teaspoon vanilla and a pinch of stevia powder and whisk until thick. You can also buy canned coconut cream and stir in vanilla and stevia. I love to plunk a tablespoon into a shot of coffee and then hit the gym afterward!

PROTEIN POWDER

Whey protein is another gray area in the dairy department, and it becomes black and white for some people. If you are not dairy sensitive, you can enjoy some whey protein smoothies a few times per week, but it must be a high-quality version. You will need to look for a minimally processed, nondenatured whey from grass-fed cows that hasn't been subjected to high temperatures when manufactured. Steer clear of any whey protein that has been subjected to cross-flow filtration, microfiltration, ultrafiltration, hydrolyzation, or ion-exchange methods, which denature the original proteins. The vast majority of whey proteins available use high-heat pasteurization. High heat does irreversible damage to the majority of the components of milk and may cause intolerance even in individuals who have no history of milk allergies.

A quality whey supplement will contain lactoferrin, immunoglobulins, serum albumin, active peptides, and growth factors, which are the most important proteins present.

Whey is a quality source of protein, but bear in mind that drinking your calories will trigger a higher insulin response. Postworkout is an ideal time to consume whey, for this very reason. Also bear in mind that although whey is a component of dairy, it's still a processed food, so use it judiciously. The same goes for goat's protein, which is derived from goat's milk. I recommend Action Whey by Emerald Essentials (see Recommended Products, page 268)—it is cold-processed whey from the raw milk of grass-fed cows.

If your whey is sweetened, make sure that it is plain, sweetened with stevia, or with xylitol for occasional use.

Coffee

Although our Paleo ancestors didn't consume coffee or much caffeine, I believe it can still be a healthy part of a Paleo diet. If you're not a regular coffee drinker, I wouldn't advocate that you start, but if it works for you, and you're having only one cup per day, then keep on rocking. The most important piece of advice I have is to drink organic coffee, since regular coffee is a concentrated source of pesticides. No need to take on extra toxins in your body, right? The best time to drink coffee is right before your workout, because it can enhance your performance and endurance. (While you're at it, maybe you should have it before sex too!)

Booze

I admit it: I've curtailed my martini drinking days in favor of fermented grapes. And if you're going to drink booze, red wine is the best one for your health. Spanish wines are richest in antioxidants because the grapes are grown at higher altitudes and need a thicker skin to protect themselves from being closer to the sun. This means a higher antioxidant content for you and me. Our Paleo ancestors consumed small amounts of alcohol on occasion, in the form of fermented fruits; we've since taken things up a notch by fermenting grapes and drinking higher amounts of alcohol at one sitting. Use alcohol within the parameters of a cheat meal (one to two drinks max). If not, it's like hitting the pause button on your body's ability to burn fat.

What About Soy?

So glad you asked!

The ploy of soy is a big problem. So many health benefits have been made in the name of soy. I used to eat a lot of soy products—tofu, soybeans, tempeh, soy milk—but through the years I have unearthed some hard truths that made me think twice about consuming soy.

- Soy lacks methionine, an essential amino acid required to build muscle. I guess that's why you don't see a lot of vegetarian bodybuilders.
- Soy suppresses thyroid function because it contains phytoestrogens that can disrupt hormonal balance.
- Soybeans are high in phytic acid, which, in large amounts, can block the uptake of essential minerals such as calcium, magnesium, copper, iron, and zinc in the intestinal tract.
- Soybeans are new to the food chain of modern man; it wasn't eaten in Paleolithic times. Many people are allergic to soy and suffer with extreme gas and bloating from it. If you have any type of autoimmune condition, especially colitis or celiac disease, remove soy from your diet immediately.
- Soy is high in the amino acid arginine and can exacerbate cold sores and herpes outbreaks.

If you're trying to remove soy from your diet, know that it is often a wolf in sheep's clothing and can have many aliases. Food manufacturers are less likely to list the three-letter word *soy* than to use a technical term such as "textured vegetable protein" (TVP), "textured plant protein," "hydrolyzed vegetable protein" (HVP), "vegetable oil," and "MSG" (monosodium glutamate). Ingredient lists also include words such as *vegetable oil, vegetable broth, bouillon, natural flavor,* or *monoglyceride*—which may or may not come from soy. Your guess is as good as mine. Plus, most soybeans are GMOs, which means that they can upset gut function as well.

Many studies have shown that traditionally fermented soy—the form popular in Asian cultures—aids in preventing and reducing a variety of diseases, including certain forms of heart disease and cancers. But just to be safe, I recommend using these products as condiments. These include miso, natto, tempeh, soy sauces, and fermented tofu. The fermentation process stops the effect of phytic acid and increases the availability of isoflavones, which are compounds that act as phytoestrogens. The fermentation also creates probiotics and ultimately increases the quantity, availability, digestibility, and assimilation of nutrients in the body.

Camp Detox: The First Fourteen Days

Here's what you can eat during the first two weeks of Paleo Detox:

1. Meals consisting of protein, vegetables, and quality fats.
2. Determine your protein requirements (see page 77).
3. 1 serving of fruit after each workout.
4. No ingredients or foods with sugar and processed starches.
5. Caffeinated coffee only before workouts; green tea the rest of the day.
6. 3 green drinks per day: drink freshly juiced greens or mix 1 tablespoon PaleoGreens in 8 ounces of water or add to your postworkout protein shake; I like the lemon-lime flavor on the rocks! Available at Designs for Health (800-847-8302).
7. Drinking water and staying well hydrated is a must. So drink up, buttercup! Aim for 8 to 10 glasses per day.

During this phase, your meals will be pretty simple. I suggest that you prep all your fruits and vegetables and cook and freeze some other dishes before you start Day 1. This way you'll have enough food on hand so that you can just grab your grub and go! Since your meals will be pretty simple, keep grilled chicken breasts or other meats and cut-up vegetables in the fridge. Keep your meals clean and lean so that you can get the gorgeous results you want in no time flat. The Paleo Detox includes simple recipes because I don't want you to spend a lot of time prepping and cooking five meals and snacks a day.

If, however, you want to spice things up and be a little more ambitious, you can certainly try the recipes in Paleo Reset or Paleo Chic.

As you move into Paleo Reset and Paleo Chic, there will be additional recipes and more wiggle room when it comes to carbs and starches.

You can refer to the Paleo Recipes section (page 195) for the more complex meals. Bon appétit, my sweet!

Day 1

Breakfast: 2 scrambled eggs with spinach, tomatoes, and onions, cooked in 1 tablespoon coconut oil.

Snack: 2 tablespoons almond butter on 2 celery sticks.

Lunch: 6 ounces grilled chicken breast with a spinach, tomato, cucumber, and ¼ avocado salad, dressed with 1 tablespoon each of extra-virgin olive oil and balsamic vinegar.

Snack: 2 rolled turkey slices with ¼ avocado and 1 raw carrot.

Dinner: 6 ounces grilled flank steak, roasted Brussels sprouts (Roasting Those Vegetables, page 121), and Green Salad (page 214) with 1 tablespoon each extra-virgin olive oil and balsamic vinegar.

Day 2

Breakfast: 4 ounces cooked turkey bacon with 10 almonds and 1-inch slice of cantaloupe.

Snack: 2 ounces smoked salmon slices with ¼ avocado.

Lunch: 6-ounce grilled hamburger with mustard and sauerkraut, 10 spears grilled asparagus with sautéed onions. (In small skillet, sauté ½ chopped onion in 1 teaspoon extra-virgin olive oil until translucent.)

Snack: 2 large hard-boiled eggs with 10 almonds.

Dinner: Turkey chili: In large skillet, brown 1 pound ground turkey in 1 tablespoon coconut oil. Add 32-ounce jar organic tomato sauce. Simmer 30 minutes and remove from heat. Stir in spinach leaves from 1 bunch, cover, and let steam for 2 minutes. Serve chili hot. Serves 4.

ROASTING THOSE VEGETABLES

One of my favorite ways to prepare and serve vegetables is to roast them. It's the best way to coax the most flavor out of Brussels sprouts, winter or summer squash, fennel, green beans, broccoli, cauliflower, and sweet potatoes, with minimal effort on your part. These crisp treats are delicious right from the oven, at room temperature, or from the fridge for a snack.

Cut vegetables into bite-size pieces. In a large bowl, toss the vegetables with 1 tablespoon extra-virgin olive oil and ½ teaspoon sea salt; you can add ¼ teaspoon freshly ground pepper as well. Arrange the vegetables in a single layer on a baking sheet. Roast at 400°F for 20 to 30 minutes, turning once at 10 to 15 minutes, until done to your liking.

Day 3

Breakfast: 3 links turkey sausage with sliced tomatoes.

Snack: 3-ounce can wild Alaskan salmon mixed with 1 teaspoon extra-virgin olive oil and 2 teaspoons cider vinegar. Serve atop cucumber slices.

Lunch: Lettuce roll-ups: 4 ounces chicken slices topped with 1 teaspoon mustard and wrapped in romaine lettuce leaves.

Snack: Handful of nuts and 2 ounces beef jerky.

Dinner: 6 ounces grilled tilapia with kale chips and Green Salad (page 214) with 1 tablespoon each extra-virgin olive oil and balsamic vinegar.

Day 4

Breakfast: 3 slices turkey bacon with 1 sliced tomato and ¼ avocado.
Snack: 2 ounces grilled chicken and asparagus spears.
Lunch: 6 ounces grilled, baked, or poached wild salmon on a bed
of cooked spinach, topped with juice of ½ lemon and
1 tablespoon extra-virgin olive oil.
Snack: 2 ounces sliced turkey with tomato slices.
Dinner: ⅓ pound ground bison, sautéed with onion powder, garlic
powder, and fresh parsley; 2 cups steamed broccoli.

Day 5

Breakfast: 3 large eggs scrambled in 1 teaspoon butter with side of
Steamed Spinach (page 236).
Snack: 2 ounces lean beef slices, carrot sticks.
Lunch: Large mixed Green Salad (page 214) topped with
1 tablespoon each extra-virgin olive oil and balsamic
vinegar, 6 ounces grilled chicken breast.
Snack: 2 cups steamed shrimp and cucumber slices.
Dinner: 6 ounces baked pork chop and 2 cups roasted cauliflower
(Roasting Those Vegetables, page 121).

Day 6

Breakfast: 3-egg omelet with mushrooms, onions, and peppers
cooked in 1 tablespoon butter.
Snack: 3-ounce can tuna with sliced tomatoes and cucumbers.
Lunch: ⅓ pound ground turkey sautéed with onion and garlic
powder and 2 cups roasted Brussels sprouts (Roasting
Those Vegetables, page 121).
Snack: Celery stalks with 1 tablespoon almond butter.
Dinner: 6-ounce grilled flank steak and 10 asparagus spears.

Day 7

Breakfast: 2 links organic chicken sausage and 10 cherry tomatoes, halved.

Snack: 2 poached large eggs and 1 cup steamed green beans.

Lunch: 6 ounces grilled chicken on lettuce, cucumbers, and tomatoes dressed with 2 tablespoons balsamic vinegar and 1 tablespoon extra-virgin olive oil.

Snack: 2 ounces smoked salmon and tomato slices.

Dinner: 6 ounces grilled tilapia and 2 cups grilled vegetables.

Day 8

Breakfast: 6 ounces steak with spinach and mushrooms cooked in 1 teaspoon butter.

Snack: Handful of almonds and 3-ounce can tuna.

Lunch: 6-ounce grilled chicken breast on lettuce, tomatoes, and cucumbers dressed with 1 tablespoon each balsamic vinegar and extra-virgin olive oil.

Snack: 2 ounces sliced turkey with ¼ avocado.

Dinner: 6 ounces grilled salmon with 2 cups grilled mixed vegetables.

Day 9

Breakfast: 2 hard-boiled large eggs with ¼ avocado and 1 sliced tomato.

Snack: 3-ounce can of salmon with 1 bunch sautéed spinach.

Lunch: Baked 4-ounce chicken drumstick with 10 spears steamed asparagus drizzled with 1 teaspoon each extra-virgin olive oil and lemon juice.

Snack: 2 ounces beef jerky with 1 cup kale chips.

Dinner: 4 ounces flank steak, 2 cups Steamed Broccoli (page 235) drizzled with 2 teaspoons each extra-virgin olive oil and lemon juice.

Day 10

Breakfast: 3 slices turkey bacon with 5 pecan halves and
1 clementine.
Snack: 2 celery sticks with 1 tablespoon almond butter.
Lunch: 6 ounces roasted salmon with tomatoes and onions.
Snack: 2 ounces sliced turkey with ¼ avocado.
Dinner: 6-ounce baked pork chop with 2 cups roasted Brussels
sprouts (Roasting Those Vegetables, page 121).

Day 11

Breakfast: 3 large scrambled eggs with cherry tomatoes and
10 cashews.
Snack: 2 turkey slices with 1 cup each raw carrots and bell pepper
slices.
Lunch: 4 ounces grilled flank steak on butter lettuce with 1
tablespoon each balsamic vinegar and extra-virgin olive oil.
Snack: 2 tablespoons cashew butter and 2 celery stalks.
Dinner: 2 cups grilled shrimp (roughly ½ pound) with 2 cups
roasted cauliflower (Roasting Those Vegetables, page 121).

Day 12

Breakfast: 2 links cooked turkey sausage with 1 sliced heirloom
tomato and 2 tablespoons pistachios.
Snack: 2 large hard-boiled eggs with ¼ avocado.
Lunch: Taco-less salad: Sauté 4 ounces ground turkey in
2 teaspoons coconut oil; place atop a salad of sliced
tomatoes and onions.
Snack: 2 ounces beef jerky and 10 almonds.
Dinner: 6 ounces grilled salmon with 1 sliced and grilled zucchini.

Day 13

Breakfast: 3 ounces smoked salmon with cucumber slices and ¼ avocado.

Snack: 2 turkey slices rolled around ¼ sliced avocado.

Lunch: ½ cup chicken salad inside a hollowed-out bell pepper. Chop up a cooked chicken breast and toss with 1 tablespoon each extra-virgin olive oil and apple cider vinegar. Spoon mixture inside bell pepper.

Snack: 2 carrots dipped into 2 tablespoons tahini.

Dinner: 6 ounces grilled flank steak with mushrooms and onions sautéed in 1 tablespoon butter.

Day 14

Breakfast: 3-egg omelet with spinach and mushrooms cooked in 1 teaspoon butter.

Snack: 2 turkey slices with ¼ avocado.

Lunch: 5-ounce grilled buffalo burger topped with thick-cut tomato slices and ¼ chopped avocado, wrapped in 2 romaine lettuce leaves.

Snack: 1 tablespoon almond butter and carrot and celery sticks.

Dinner: 5 large skillet-seared scallops with 2 cups kale chips and Green Salad (page 214) dressed with 1 tablespoon each olive oil and lemon juice.

Analyze This . . .

As you work through the three Paleo phases of *Cavewomen Don't Get Fat*, keep in mind that your body has different needs than those of your friends. These are overall *guidelines* that will fluctuate based on your training schedule, stress levels, sleep, hormones, and all the other pieces of our lives that often require fine-tuning. You may need to tweak these plans to better suit your needs. I'm not a believer in counting calories, but it's essential to be in the proper zone for your body to achieve proper fat loss. If you're training with heavy weights four days per week, you'll need to eat more calories to compensate for your caloric expenditure during workouts and the fat burned after workouts and to preserve lean muscle mass. But if you're trying to lose body fat, then you can shave off about 300 calories per day. The good news is that once you eliminate carbs, you'll do this naturally. Eating this way, it is possible for women to gain lean muscle mass while simultaneously losing body fat.

CHAPTER 9

Paleo Reset

Once you finish the fourteen-day Paleo Detox, you're ready for the Paleo Reset, which loosens the reins a bit and allows you to enjoy more carbs but still enables you to continue on your fat-loss journey. The great news is that you can still expect one to two pounds of fat loss a week. This phase balances your hormones and tackles body fat. Stay on this plan until your body fat percentage goal is reached. How long is that? It all depends on your individual biochemistry and your commitment to eating Paleo.

The Cheat Meal

The Paleo Reset phase allows you to have one cheat meal each week to help reset your leptin level (see page 102) and prevent you from becoming weight-loss resistant. But before you dive headfirst into a bowl of chocolate pudding, let's take a moment to discuss some logistics. True, cavewomen could not really cheat on their diets because all the sweets and processed foods we now have access to did not exist at the time. (And, accessibility to food in general was inconsistent for hunter-gatherers, making actual consistency of meals more of an issue than anything else.) There was no cake to cheat with, no soda to slug back, and certainly no unlimited access to all things sweet. So why do I allow it on the Paleo Chic plan? Because we do live in a world with cake, and I'm not going to tell you that you can never enjoy another bite in your life. But I am going to tell you that there's a fine line between indulging and overindulging, and gorging yourself on a weekend bender can set you right back to your starting point.

There is also a case to be made for not cheating with junk food, but, instead, increasing your total quantity of food. Reestablishing your leptin level is less about junk food than the total quantity of food. So instead of pigging out on junk food, you can increase the volume of food you consume (think double portions), and you will still achieve the desired effect. You can also cheat every other week to really up your fat-loss game.

So respect the cheat meal. Remember that it is not a license to ill but simply another tool in your belt for coaxing along the weight loss process. Your goal is not to overstuff yourself and wake up with a hangover the next day; it's to satisfy a craving and then get back to business.

Dieting can lower your leptin levels, and severely limiting your carbohydrates for more than a couple weeks can raise your cortisol levels. Cheat meal to the rescue! Throwing your metabolism a curveball will prevent your leptin from getting out of line and keep your stress hormones in check. We rarely have the opportunity to trick our bodies into weight loss, but a planned cheat meal can achieve just that. Plus, it will keep you psychologically fulfilled and allow you to enjoy your favorite foods on occasion. Done correctly, the cheat meal can add back some sensuality to your eating experience and create what I consider the ultimate bliss: a life lived in balance.

A cheat meal is a necessary part of fat loss. Strategically planning a cheat meal will boost your metabolism and reach the pleasure centers in the deepest parts of your brain. And when you have a craving for a piece of pizza or a slice of chocolate cake, knowing that you will be able to enjoy them in just a few days keeps you honest. We all need a carrot—or a cupcake—dangled in front of us to keep us motivated. The cheat meal does just that.

As you get leaner, you can incorporate two cheat meals per week to keep your body guessing. Don't abuse your privileges, though, or you won't see the benefits you've worked so hard to gain—or lose.

What does a cheat meal look like? Allow me to show you the path of enlightenment:

Hamburger and French fries, chocolate chip cookie
Pancakes with butter and syrup and sausages
Enchiladas with beans and rice, sour cream, guacamole, and
    cheese, and a beer
Cheese ravioli with a glass of wine
Sushi and sake
Bagel with cream cheese and smoked salmon
Pork dumplings, shrimp fried rice, broccoli with brown sauce,
    and green tea ice cream

Tips When Eating Your Cheat Meal

- Carbohydrates will raise your leptin levels and, to a lesser extent, insulin. So keep your fat intake low if you are eating a higher-carbohydrate meal. Your insulin levels will be high enough as it is; adding fat with a storage hormone will not give you the desired results.
- No need to count calories, but exercise the boundaries of decency!
- Experiment for a bit to see how your body reacts to your cheat meals. You will have to see how this shakes out. Some women can tolerate gluten on occasion; other babes blow up like balloons after eating a sandwich. How your body

responds really depends on your genetic makeup. So if a cheat meal that includes gluten doesn't work for you, keep your carb choices clean and gluten-free.

- Time your cheat meal accordingly. In a perfect world, we would have our cheat meals immediately following a workout, when our insulin sensitivity is highest. At that point in time, your muscles are primed and ready for a hot night out in carb town, and you'll be less likely to store the carbohydrates you do eat as fat. Most women like to save their cheat meals for the weekend, when they're more likely to go out to eat. Whenever you do, just have fun and revel in the pleasure of delicious foods. I love to save up a cheat meal for a date night out so I can loosen the reins a bit. I'll have a glass of wine, eat a hearty meal that's usually gluten-free—for instance, steak, risotto, and spinach—and I'll have some spoonfuls of dessert. Overall, though, I'd much rather drink booze than eat sugar!

- Go all out, but don't blow it. I must put in a small disclaimer here. The goal of the cheat meal is to reset your leptin levels, not gain back everything you worked so hard to lose. You can't eat unlimited amounts of food and not gain weight. So unless you are lifting heavy weights and training to be a superhero in an action movie, you are probably going to need to limit the amounts of food—and, dare I say it, calories—you are eating in your cheat meal. Everyone wants to find the dietary loophole that will enable them to toss accountability out the window, but I'm afraid no one's discovered it yet! So go and enjoy your cheat meal, but don't make it a 2,000-calorie event, either.

- Make sure that you work out and drink plenty of water the day of your cheat meal, to minimize the bloating from a food hangover the next day.

Is a Cheat Meal for You?

The thing to remember about a cheat meal is that when it works, it works beautifully, but it does require serious discipline and self-control. There have been times when it took me three days for my sugar cravings to die down after my cheat meal. It was oh-so mentally challenging to stay on track during those three days. If the Paleo way of eating is completely new to you, it may be too challenging to dip your toe in the pool for a night without being able to take a long swim. You have to have an honest conversation with yourself and figure out what works best for you.

You may want to take a bit more time to get the Paleo way of eating under your shrinking belt and get hold of your blood sugar swings before you reintroduce the foods that got you into trouble in the first place. If you feel the cheat meal is going to send you back to your old eating habits, then keep your cheat meals gluten-free and clean, and work within those parameters until you're ready to make the leap.

Why Are Certain Foods So Hard to Give Up?

Food addictions are not just a psychological issue, they're also a physical issue. Processed foods fire up dopamine receptors in the brain, making us immediately crave more. Some of us are more sensitive to these effects than others, and the effect on the brain is like smack to a junkie. Eating processed foods can have the same outcome. Bear in mind that it can take at least seven days to quell your sugar cravings and up to a month to recover fully from junk-food cravings once you clean them out from your diet. That's normal, so cut yourself some slack and just go with it. Knowing what to expect is half the battle. The rewards will be the improvements you see in your body and feel in your mind.

Change Is a Process, and the Process Is the Goal

Cavewomen Don't Get Fat is all about changing your lifestyle and changing the way you eat. And that means you have to change the way you live. And *that* means your lifestyle doesn't affect just you but also everyone around you. That's not a bad thing, mind you; leading by example can help get others on board. ("Wow, you look great! Really? Maybe I should become a cavewoman too!") For most of us, though, change can be terrifying. Food is such a complicated topic, and often the strongest memories we have of food go back to our childhood.

What you need to take away from this is that the past is a place of reference, not a place of residence. Letting go of old attachments to foods that stand in the way of your goals is the best way to literally clear your plate for new opportunities. Healing requires change. Once we can let go of the past and start to change our bodies, we wonder why we didn't choose this path sooner.

Take Ownership over Your Actions

If you're anything like me, then you don't have much willpower or self-control. It takes a phenomenal amount of effort on my part to resist my mother's homemade cookies. And I never want to feel guilty after I eat them, either. So I build a cheat meal into visits to my parents' house so that I can have a couple cookies and not only not feel bad about it but feel like I'm doing my body a favor!

Let's talk for a moment about discipline, which is different than control. Most of us struggle to control what we eat, but it's discipline that will help you reach your goals.

According to my friend Jade Teta, author of *The New Me Diet: Eat More, Work Out Less, and Actually Lose Weight While You Rest*, control is an illusion, because we rarely have that kind of power. Discipline, on the other hand, involves making a conscious choice. When we set goals and reach them, we are making conscious choices to take responsibility and make certain things happen. Getting to the gym, shopping for and preparing healthful meals, going to bed on time, and spending quality time with family and friends are all conscious choices that we make. When we choose foods and exercises that fall within our goals, we naturally achieve the art of discipline. The beauty of discipline is that it can evolve organically when we have all our ducks lined up in a row. And by making great choices for ourselves, we regain self-control. Make sense?

If you can't change your eating habits overnight, it's more important to acknowledge the space you're in and go forth at your own rate than it is to take on too many changes at once and set yourself up for failure. We exist within the parameters we set for ourselves. If something that I suggest doesn't feel authentic for you when you're overhauling your eating habits, then take your time and figure out what works for you. Opening yourself up to change happens when you are ready; no sooner than that. It's not about judgment, self-criticism, or self-flagellation; it's about self-acceptance and hunkering down to get the job done.

Paleo Reset

This phase balances your hunger hormones and tackles body fat. Stay on this plan until your body fat percentage goal is reached. Here's what you're going to do:

- Reintroduce one complex starch per day, such as sweet potato or winter squash, either as your postworkout meal or at dinner to facilitate quality sleep. The best time to eat your favorite carbs is within thirty minutes after finishing your workout. Following a workout, these carbs spike your insulin

level, which creates a metabolic surge that can help you build
more muscle.

- Continue to eat protein and vegetable-based meals every day.
- Weekly cheat meal: a "normal" dinner, 4 ounces of wine, and
  dessert, or a double portion of your meal, combats metabolic
  plateaus. You'll burn more fat the next day. To your salad with
  goat cheese, filet mignon with a baked potato and butter,
  you can add red wine and a slice of chocolate cake.
- Drink caffeinated coffee only before workouts to spike
  insulin and cortisol production, which burns more fat and
  helps build muscle. Drink green tea all day.
- Green drinks 2 times per day.
- Hydrate by drinking 8 to 10 glasses of water each day.

All of the recipes make 1 serving unless otherwise noted. Recipes can be found starting on page 195.

Day 1

Breakfast: Vegetable Omelet (page 197)
Snack: 2 ounces sliced turkey breast with ¼ avocado.
Lunch: 4 ounces grilled chicken and a salad: 2 cups raw spinach, 1
        sliced tomato, and ½ cucumber dressed with 1 tablespoon
        each balsamic vinegar and olive oil.
Snack: Ten almonds and 3-ounce can water-packed tuna.
Dinner: Turkey Meatballs with Spaghetti Squash and Steamed
        Broccoli (page 237).

Day 2

Breakfast: Leftover turkey meatballs and sliced bell pepper.
Snack: 2 ounces beef jerky with 1 tablespoon almond butter.
Lunch: 6 ounces Grilled Wild Alaskan Salmon and Spinach Salad
        (page 221).

Snack: Chicken-Vegetable Soup (page 254).

Dinner: Skirt Steak with Roasted Asparagus, Sweet Potato, and Onion (page 240).

Day 3

Breakfast: 3 ounces smoked wild salmon on tomato slices topped with ¼ avocado.

Snack: 1 cup steamed shrimp (about 6 ounces) with ¼ cup tomato sauce.

Lunch: Cajun Baked Pork Chops (page 219) with Steamed Broccoli (page 235).

Snack: 2 hard-boiled eggs with handful of almonds.

Dinner: Stir-Fried Chicken and Vegetables (page 233).

Day 4

Breakfast: Tropical Smoothie (page 207).

Snack: Avocado Turkey Boat (page 257).

Lunch: Apple-Walnut Chicken Salad (page 211).

Snack: 2 large hard-boiled eggs with sliced veggies.

Dinner: Turkey-Vegetable Lasagna (page 238).

Day 5

Breakfast: 2 turkey sausages cooked in 1 teaspoon coconut oil, 1 sliced bell pepper, ½ cup raw cashews.

Snack: Smoked Salmon and Red Pepper Roll-Ups (page 258).

Lunch: Lamb Chops and Broccoli Rabe (page 220).

Snack: Celery stalks with 2 tablespoons almond butter.

Dinner: 2 Stuffed Peppers (page 245) with tossed Green Salad (page 214).

Day 6

Breakfast: Grilled organic chicken sausages with sautéed spinach.
Snack: Crabmeat-Cucumber Salad (page 256).
Lunch: Buffalo Chicken Salad (page 223) with tossed Green Salad (page 214).
Snack: Piña Colada Smoothie (page 206).
Dinner: Filet Mignon and Broccoli Rabe (page 243).

Day 7

Breakfast: Creamsicle Smoothie (page 205).
Snack: 3 ounces canned salmon on cucumber slices.
Lunch: Grilled Skirt Steak with Spinach, Cranberries, and Walnuts Salad (page 215).
Snack: ¼ cup dried coconut chunks and ¼ cup nuts.
Dinner: Coconut Shrimp with Sesame Bok Choy (page 250).

Day 8

Breakfast: Sun-Dried Tomato-Pesto Omelet (page 197).
Snack: 3 ounces organic beef jerky with carrot and celery sticks.
Lunch: Twice-Baked Sweet Potato Skins with Bison, Spinach, and Turkey Bacon (page 219).
Snack: Handful of almonds and sliced carrot sticks.
Dinner: Pesto Chicken and Roasted Broccoli (page 228).

Day 9

Breakfast: Top thick-cut heirloom tomatoes with 4 ounces smoked salmon and sliced ½ avocado.
Snack: Pumpkin Pie Smoothie (page 206).

Lunch:	Roasted Chicken Breasts with Arugula and Fennel Salad (page 209).
Snack:	2 tablespoons almond butter on 2 celery stalks, topped with 5 raisins each.
Dinner:	Grilled Rosemary-Garlic Shrimp with Grilled Vegetables (page 251).

Day 10

Breakfast:	Steak with avocado and tomatoes. In small skillet, sauté 6-ounce steak in 2 teaspoons clarified butter. Top with sliced ½ avocado and large sliced tomato.
Snack:	Sliced apple with 2 tablespoons natural almond butter.
Lunch:	Curried Chicken Salad (page 213).
Snack:	4 ounces turkey slices with red pepper slices.
Dinner:	Grilled Wild Salmon with Pesto (page 246).

Day 11

Breakfast:	Brownie Surprise (page 205).
Snack:	4 slices ham wrapped around 4 asparagus stalks.
Lunch:	Lamb and Greek Salad (page 220).
Snack:	3-ounce can tuna, carrot and celery sticks.
Dinner:	Pecan-Crusted Chicken with Sautéed Asparagus and Butternut Squash Soup (page 232).

Day 12

Breakfast:	Big Breakfast (page 203).
Snack:	Watermelon, Avocado, and Hearts of Palm Salad (page 259).
Lunch:	Taco Salad (page 214).

Snack: Smoked Salmon, Fennel, and Dill Salad (page 259).
Dinner: Roasted Chicken and Green Beans (page 227).

Day 13

Breakfast: Vegetable Omelet (page 197).
Snack: Tuna Salad (page 262) on tomato slices.
Lunch: Grilled Skirt Steak and Beet Salad (page 216).
Snack: Turkey Pepper Open-Faced Sandwich (page 262).
Dinner: Almond-Crusted Tilapia and Sweet Potato Mash (page 248).

Day 14

Breakfast: PB & J Smoothie (page 206).
Snack: 2 large hard-boiled eggs with sliced cucumbers and tomatoes.
Lunch: Skirt Steak with Guasaca Sauce (page 216).
Snack: ½ grapefruit with 3 ounces smoked salmon.
Dinner: Zucchini Pasta with Meat Sauce (page 244).

CHAPTER 10

Paleo Chic

This is where the rubber meets the road, and you learn the level of carb tolerance that works for your body. Stay on this plan as long as you are within 3 to 5 percent of your body fat ideal; if you exceed this, drop back to Paleo Reset until your goal is reached. If you're eating two starches per day and one cheat meal per week, and your body fat remains within a consistent range, then you've hit your metabolic stride and can stay on this plan. If your exercise falls by the wayside and/or your body fat comes creeping back up again, you can hit the metabolic reset button by revisiting the Paleo Reset guidelines for another two weeks. Bear in mind that stress, sleep, consistency of exercise and eating, and life in general can all challenge you and your body to stay on track. But self-regulating your carb intake accordingly will make you the mistress of your own metabolic domain.

- Enjoy one or two complex starches per day, anytime, depending on your tolerance of carbs.
- Continue protein- and vegetable-based meals prepared with quality fats.
- Weekly cheat meal: one to two indulgence meals per week

that can include a glass of wine, and a "normal" dinner and dessert, or a double portion of your meal.

- Caffeine is still allowed, but coffee only *before* workouts; green tea throughout the day.
- Green drink once a day.
- Drink plenty of water and stay well hydrated throughout the day.

All of the recipes make 1 serving unless otherwise noted. Recipes can be found starting on page 197.

Day 1

Breakfast: Banana Boom Protein Smoothie (page 204).
Snack: Apple slices with 2 tablespoons almond butter.
Lunch: Taco Salad (page 214).
Snack: 2 large hard-boiled eggs with avocado slices.
Dinner: Pepper Steak with Peppers and Onions (page 243).

Day 2

Breakfast: 4-egg white omelet with sautéed veggies and side of cantaloupe.
Snack: 2 ounces grilled chicken slices with spinach.
Lunch: Southwestern Turkey Burgers (page 213) and Green Salad (page 214).
Snack: ½ cup mixed berries with 1 tablespoon almond butter.
Dinner: Sweet Potato–Crusted Wild Salmon (page 246) with grilled zucchini and Green Salad.

Day 3

Breakfast: 4 ounces smoked Alaskan salmon with 1 cup mixed berries.
Snack: Chicken, Avocado, and Walnut Salad (page 258).
Lunch: Paleo Chicken Fingers and Zucchini Sticks (page 210).

Snack: 4 ounces beef jerky with 2 carrots.
Dinner: Cajun Catfish, Mashed Parsnips and Apples, and Roasted
          Brussels Sprouts (page 247).

Day 4

Breakfast: Eggs and Chorizo Scramble (page 198).
Snack: Ants on a Log (page 258).
Lunch: Apple-Walnut Chicken Salad (page 211).
Snack: Apple Chips and a handful of almonds.
Dinner: Sesame Seared Tuna (page 249) with Seaweed Salad
          (page 250).

Day 5

Breakfast: Scrambled Eggs Topped with Avocado and Salsa (page 199).
Snack: You're Makin' Me Bananas Smoothie (page 207).
Lunch: Grilled Chicken, Spinach, and Strawberry Salad (page 212).
Snack: ½ cup Trail Mix (page 264).
Dinner: Turkey Chili and Steamed Spinach (page 235).

Day 6

Breakfast: Smoked Salmon Egg Scramble (page 199).
Snack: Chicken-Endive Boat (page 264).
Lunch: Chili-Seared Sea Scallops with Sautéed Watercress
          (page 222).
Snack: Turkey Avocado Roll-Ups (page 264).
Dinner: Fish Tacos (page 249).

Day 7

Breakfast: Paleo Blueberry Pancakes (page 200).
Snack: Berry Blast Smoothie (page 204).

Lunch: Lamb Chops and Broccoli Rabe (page 220).
Snack: Gorgeous Coconut Protein Bars (page 265).
Dinner: Spaghetti Squash with Italian Chicken Sausage and
             Steamed Broccoli (page 234).

Day 8

Breakfast: Spinach Frittata (page 200) and ½ cup mixed berries.
Snack: Mojito Shrimp Salad (page 260).
Lunch: Grilled Steak Salad with Tangerines and Almonds (page 217).
Snack: 4 ounces smoked salmon and 1 cup melon.
Dinner: Stir-Fried Chicken and Vegetables (page 233) and
             Gazpacho (page 261).

Day 9

Breakfast: Chocolate-Strawberry Smoothie (page 205).
Snack: Deviled Guacamole Eggs (page 263).
Lunch: Chef's Salad (page 212).
Snack: Paleo Dip with Vegetables (page 255).
Dinner: "Bruschetta" Chicken, Roasted Acorn Squash, and
             Sautéed Asparagus (page 229).

Day 10

Breakfast: Steak and Eggs with Tomatoes (page 201).
Snack: Bacon-Wrapped Dates (page 255).
Lunch: Salmon Burgers (page 224) and Green Salad (page 214).
Snack: Gorgeous Almond Protein Bars (page 265).
Dinner: Lettuce Wrap Turkey Tacos and Butternut Squash Soup
             (page 237).

Day 11

Breakfast: Almond Butter Dreams Smoothie (page 204).
Snack: 2 hard-boiled eggs with sliced carrots, celery, and cucumbers.
Lunch: Apple-Walnut Chicken Salad (page 211).
Snack: Salmon Salad over cucumber slices (page 262).
Dinner: Cucumber Sushi and Wasabi Mashed "Potatoes" (page 252).

Day 12

Breakfast: Crustless Mini-Quiche (page 202) with melon slices.
Snack: 5 shrimp with sliced cucumber and avocado.
Lunch: Crab Cakes with Paleo Aïoli (page 224).
Snack: Paleo Fruit Bars (page 266).
Dinner: Skirt Steak with Chimichurri Sauce, Cherry Tomatoes, and Sweet Potato Skewers (page 241).

Day 13

Breakfast: Eggs Benedict with Orange Slices (page 201).
Snack: Shrimp Ceviche (page 261).
Lunch: Burgers and Sweet Potato Fries (page 218).
Snack: Crabmeat-Stuffed Mushrooms (page 256).
Dinner: Chicken Rolled with Broccoli Rabe and Sun-Dried Tomatoes (page 231).

Day 14

Breakfast: Banana-Walnut Pancakes with Turkey Sausage (page 203).
Snack: Grilled Shrimp Skewers (page 260).
Lunch: Citrus Tilapia Salad (page 223).
Snack: Sliced carrots and cucumbers and ½ cup mixed nuts.
Dinner: Mama's Sunday Meatballs and Spaghetti Squash (page 239).

Clean Cheats

When you're dying for a sweet and have a cheat meal coming up, try any of these lurvely Paleo sweets for a clean cheat! Bear in mind that a clean cheat satisfies your sweet tooth but remains within the parameters of gluten and dairy-free Paleo eating. It still constitutes a cheat, but you may not feel as bad after eating it. A dirty cheat encompasses an all-out blitz where food rules are suspended for the meal. You decide which one will rock your world (in a good way) and enable you to get back on track the next day.

WATERMELON ICE POPS

Serves 6–8 (depending on the size of your molds)

4 cups watermelon chunks

3 fresh mint leaves or 1 mint tea bag, steeped in 2 cups water

Puree watermelon in food processor. Combine mint water with watermelon. Place mixture in popsicle molds (I use stainless steel or silicone molds) and freeze.

CHOCOLATE-TOPPED MACAROONS

Makes 20

8 ounces shredded
    unsweetened coconut
3 large egg whites

¼ cup erythritol powder or
    stevia powder
2 teaspoons vanilla extract
4 ounces dark chocolate

Preheat oven to 350°F. Line baking sheet with parchment paper. In large bowl, whisk together egg whites with sugar substitute until well combined. Add vanilla and coconut, and stir until well combined. Shape batter into golf-ball-sized balls. Arrange on a baking sheet and bake until tops become golden brown; approximately 15 minutes. Remove from oven and cool. While they are baking, melt chocolate over low heat in double boiler. Dip macaroons in chocolate or drizzle on top. Refrigerate until chocolate is set and serve.

CHOCOLATE-COVERED STRAWBERRIES

Serves 6

4 ounces dark chocolate
1 dozen large strawberries

Heat chocolate in double boiler over medium heat. Keep stirring chocolate until melted. Dip strawberries in chocolate until fully coated. Place strawberries on baking sheet lined with wax paper. Refrigerate for 2 hours or until chocolate is set.

COCONUT BROWNIES

Makes 16

1 scoop chocolate protein powder

1 tablespoon cocoa powder

½ teaspoon vanilla extract

12 prunes, pitted

1 tablespoon almond butter

3 tablespoons almond flour

2 tablespoons coconut milk

2 teaspoons shredded coconut

Place protein powder, cocoa powder, vanilla extract, prunes, and almond butter in food processor. Blend until smooth and creamy. Add almond flour and coconut milk. Transfer to bowl and fold in shredded coconut. Scrape batter into an 8 x 8-inch pan and spread evenly. Refrigerate for 30 minutes before cutting and serving.

AVOCADO-CHOCOLATE PUDDING

Serves 4

1 avocado, cut up

1 banana

2 tablespoons honey

½ cup cocoa powder

2 tablespoons coconut oil, at room temperature

1 teaspoon vanilla extract

Place all ingredients into blender or food processor. Blend until mixture thickens into pudding consistency. Divide among four ramekins. Chill for 1 hour and serve.

GRILLED BANANAS

Serves 2

2 bananas, quartered
1 tablespoon coconut oil
or clarified butter

1 teaspoon ground
cinnamon
2 teaspoons raw honey

Brush coconut oil on bananas and sprinkle with cinnamon. Grill or skillet-fry bananas for about 2 to 4 minutes on each side. Drizzle with honey and serve warm.

FEED YOUR BELLY

It takes more than just food to feed your belly right; you also need to keep your gut healthy with probiotics. Probiotics are the "good" bacteria that live inside our intestinal tracts, such as lactobacillus and bifidobacteria. They keep our guts and immune systems healthy and also help us gals stay regular. Nowadays, the bacteria inside the intestinal tract are considered to be their own separate organ. These bacteria weigh about three to four pounds, amounting to billions of bacteria that populate the gut. Every day we naturally shed and turn over some of those bacteria through our bowel movements, and more colonize in their place. Both men and women have "good" bacteria and "bad" bacteria that maintain an intricate balance within the gut. Certain lifestyle factors can disrupt this delicate balance, such as stress, excessive alcohol and sugar, a low-fiber, high-sugar diet, and medications like antibiotics and oral contraceptives. A whole-foods diet rich in fiber will do your body justice and help build good bacteria. Garlic, plain yogurt (assuming that you tolerate dairy), and ground flax or chia seeds are all functional foods that can help create a healthy gut environment. And taking a probiotic supplement daily is also beneficial; see chapter 11 on supplements for more information.

Troubleshooting

So here you are, ready and prepped for your badass Paleo life. With a chicken drumstick in one hand and some dried coconut flakes in the other, you're off to the gym to lift some weights and tackle some sprints. You've been doing this for a month but haven't seen any changes in your body. Your clothes aren't any looser. You're saying, "Esther? What's going on?"

Believe me, you're not alone. Let's talk about some of the deeper reasons why you're not making the progress you'd like, and what you can do about it.

You're Toxic. Looks like it's time to hit the detox protocol, stat. Visit the toxic waist chapter (Chapter 4: Do These Toxins Make Me Look Fat?) for lifestyle changes to remove toxins from your bod. And visit a holistic MD to get tested for toxins.

You're Intolerant. Here's the great irony in eating clean: in simplifying your diet and purging processed carbs from your pantry, you will have less variety in the foods that you are eating. That means you can overexpose yourself to staples such as meat, eggs, and fish, and then develop food intolerances to those foods. Most of us don't even realize that we've sensitized our immune systems because we may not even show symptoms of intolerances. But the intolerances can cause low levels of inflammation throughout the body, disrupting the gut and immune system, and making it difficult to drop body fat. Eggs, nuts, soy, corn, wheat, and dairy are the most common allergens found in food, but at any point, you can develop allergies to innocuous foods such as parsley, blueberries, lamb, or broccoli. And the more regularly you eat a particular food, the greater the chance that you can become allergic to it. So rotate, rotate, rotate! Do not eat the same things every day; alternate your proteins, fats, fruits, and vegetables as much as possible.

If you suspect you're intolerant, you can ask your nutritionally oriented physician to help you determine what foods are the main culprits. The LEAP MRT (Lifestyle, Eating, and Performance Mediator Release Test) is a comprehensive blood panel that tests your immune system response to 120 foods and 30 different chemicals and additives. MRT is a functional live-cell analysis that identifies foods and chemicals that provoke the release of mediators that cause pain and inflammation.

You're Not Managing Your Stress. In chapter 3, I explained how stress is the underlying culprit for hormonal imbalances, heart disease, chronic ailments, and anxiety and depression. Take a good, hard look at the people you surround yourself with, and then purge anyone toxic from your life. Abusive people who suck you dry emotionally or waste your time can stress out your system and cause you to hold on to fat, especially in your midsection. Many of us are resistant to getting rid of toxic relationships or just can't do it at all. Do the best you can to keep toxic people out of your life and you'll be not only happier but also healthier.

You Need to Work Out Smarter. If you're like me, you don't have hours to spend working out. I have other things to do. So when I do, it has to be an all-out scenario. Most of us either don't understand what our bodies are capable of, or just don't like feeling like we're going to cough up a lung during a workout. But to change your body composition, you have to push your body to places you never thought possible. You will need to silence the voice inside your head that tells you to stop before your designated sets are finished. You just have to suck it up and work harder. It's not about the quantity of time you spend in the gym; it's about the quality and the intensity of your workouts. If you want to be a cavewoman, strength training is essential for maintaining muscle mass while losing body fat.

You're Overdoing Cardio. Hopping on the elliptical machine like a hamster on a wheel or taking two spin classes in a row won't make a dent in your fat loss. Excess cardio jacks up your cortisol, the hormone that instructs your belly to store excess fat and keeps your stress hormones elevated for hours after a workout. Over time, this can interfere with your insulin metabolism and adversely affect the thyroid and the adrenals. Funk that! The best forms of cardio are walking, hiking, yoga, sprinting, jumping rope, and plyometrics—explosive, fast movements that build maximum power in functional movements. If you lift weights but crave cardio, then lift them faster! Thirty minutes of sprints twice per week is plenty, and walking can be done until you can't put one foot in front of the other. Just get outdoors, enjoy the fresh air, and watch your cortisol, stress, and body fat levels fall effortlessly.

Scaling back on cardio also gives you the chance to boost your levels of growth hormone. Growth hormone stimulates growth and regeneration and supports the production of lean muscle mass. Its level is highest when we are young and growing; as we age, the level drops naturally, and we produce much less (though women do produce more than men). Some people try to prevent the effects of aging by injecting themselves with growth hormone, but eating clean foods and strength-building exercise are the best things you can do to produce the juice naturally. Sleep and exercise also play huge roles in the production and release of growth hormone. Sprinting at your maximum threshold and engaging large muscle groups during lifting sessions will give your body the greatest rise in growth hormone.

You're Eating Carbs at the Wrong Time. If your body fat is above 20 percent, chances are your body isn't as sensitive to insulin and carbs as you'd like to think. This red flag can prevent you from reaching your fitness goals. I suggest that you eat 75 to 100 grams of carbohydrates from sweet potato or winter squash (1 cup cooked) with your nightly meal or postworkout, and eat carbs from vegetable sources the rest of the day. Another option is not to eat starchy carbs for three days and then on Day 4 load up with four starch servings throughout the day and postworkout. As previously mentioned, you should eat carbs only after a workout or at your evening meal. Eating plenty of protein and fat throughout the day provides your noggin with pure, gorgeous, brain food that will keep your mental focus sharp as a tack while hammering away at your daily tasks. Then, at night, a dose of carbs will help jack up your serotonin levels so that you can relax, rest, and repair while having a delicious night's sleep. Bliss!

You're Eating Too Much Fat. Whoa, cavegirl! Esther said *what*? "I thought I could eat a lot of quality fat in my diet?" Yes, you can, if you're totally sinewy and lifting heavy weights and burning body fat like crazy. But if you're sitting on your tush all day at work and flopping down on the sofa at night to watch three or more hours of television, you're not burning as much fat as you think you are. So no, you may not snarf down 2 cups of nuts at one sitting or add a stick of butter to your steamed vegetables. Be reasonable and be accountable for what you put in your mouth. Eat 10 nuts at a time or a heaping teaspoon of nut butter. If you don't see changes in your body composition, then you'll need to eat less fat.

You're Not Eating Enough Protein. Oh, cave sister, how I can relate to this one! When I was in my twenties, I ate a bagel with cream cheese and coffee for breakfast, beans and rice or sushi for lunch, and pasta for dinner. Although I was thin at the time, I didn't have any muscle definition or any energy. Like most women, I wasn't eating enough protein. We tend to suck down whatever carbs we can get our hands on as a quick fix to battle hunger. When we crash and burn later, the whole cycle starts again. Women need to eat 1 gram of protein per pound of body weight every day. So a woman who weighs 140 pounds should eat 140 grams of protein, which equals 20 ounces of protein (there are 7 grams of protein in one ounce). This shakes out to an average of 5 ounces of protein at meals, plus another 2–3 ounces of protein at two snacks throughout the day. Protein will keep you sailing through your day with energy and will help you get lean.

You're Drinking Too Many Protein Shakes. I'm all about replenishing your body with some postworkout protein, like a shake. But some women rely on them too frequently throughout the day instead of eating real food. Drinking protein shakes while on a travel day beats eating the junk food available in airports, but don't make it a habit. If you're struggling to lose body fat, and you're having more than one shake a day, cut back. Whey protein raises the body's insulin level, which is exactly what you want to accomplish immediately following your workout. A surge of insulin will activate the release of growth hormone to help you build lean muscle. The trick is to keep that surge encapsulated within a thirty-minute window postworkout. Having a shake midafternoon will only raise your insulin level and stand in the way of your fitness goals. We also must remember that chewing and digesting food burns calories. Drinking our food requires much less work from the gut because shakes are more easily digested, so you'll burn fewer calories as a result. Chew your calories as often as you can.

You're Eating Too Much Fruit. Say it isn't so! It's easy for me to give up many foods, but fruits are a tough one for me to eliminate entirely. Yes, fruits have antioxidants, fight diseases, clean your intestines, and satisfy a sweet tooth. Most of the fruit we eat today are sugar bombs compared with the tart (and sometimes bitter) ones that our ancestors ate. They are rich in fructose, which can not only prevent you from burning fat during a workout but also lead to fat gain if you're eating too much of it. The liver processes fructose, and once the liver has reached its glycogen storage limit, excess glycogen gets converted to triglycerides and stored as body fat. So limit your fruit to 1 or 2 servings per day to get lean, and make sure you're consuming plenty of dark, deeply pigmented vegetables to reach your nutritional needs.

You've Fallen Off the Paleo Pony. Diet will dictate 80 percent of your fat loss. It also requires razor-sharp focus and self-empowerment when we make our food choices. Second in line to diet is your exercise program, which will help you maintain lean muscle mass. If you're not sticking to your clean Paleo diet, and your cheat meal has become an all-out food orgy, you can sleep twelve hours a day, exercise your heart out, and still not see results. Diet is truly that important.

You're Not Getting Enough Sleep. Sleep is a fat-loss nutrient and rules the hormonal roost. Think of sleep as a dictator of its citizens, which are your hormones. Under conditions of sleep deprivation, your insulin sensitivity decreases while your cortisol shoots up. Trying to budge your body fat under such conditions will result in a failed mission. Sleep—a long restful night's sleep of seven to nine hours—improves everything: muscle gains, appetite control, fat loss, mood, and cognitive function. So make it a priority.

What About Intermittent Fasting?

Intermittent fasting (IF) is a huge buzzword among those living the Paleo Chic lifestyle. The guidelines for IF are that you eat the same number of calories every day, but you consume those calories in fewer hours during the day. Some people choose to eat only when they are hungry and don't have their first meal until ten or eleven o'clock in the morning, while others eat only between the hours of eleven and five. The premise is that human beings evolved to survive under suboptimal conditions when food wasn't readily available, so the body is designed to fast for long periods of time.

I know some strength coaches and colleagues who find that IF works well for them and helps them maintain a lean physique. But it depends on your body composition and how you feel. Typically, pear-shaped women feel better and lose more fat with IF than apple-shaped women do, but this is not a cut-and-dry statement. Many women suffer from insomnia, anxiety, irregular periods, and hormonal imbalances as a consequence of IF. Much of the research on IF has been done on men, which isn't helpful in determining the effects it has on us girls. Out of seventy-one peer-reviewed studies on the benefits of IF, only thirteen used female subjects and those did not delve into the potential metabolic consequences of IF for a woman. My concern is that these sex-based oversights can overlook the potential damage to a woman's metabolism, fertility, adrenal fatigue, hormones, and circadian rhythms in the long run. So if you are of reproductive age and considering IF, be mindful of the potential strains it can put on your system and err on the side of caution. There isn't enough scientific evidence out there to justify fasting.

Contain Yourself!

Since you're already investing in yourself by eating the healthiest foods in the world, it's important to protect that investment by storing your food in quality containers. Stainless steel and glass containers make excellent choices, since both are chemically inert. If you must store your food in plastic containers, look for "BPA-free" on the label and use plastic containers with recycling labels numbers 1, 2, or 4, which do not contain the chemical BPA, or bisphenol A. Steer clear of the number 7 label, which often does contain BPA. I advise you not to microwave your foods, but if you must, please do so in a glass container; microwaving plastic will cause BPA and any other inert chemicals lurking around to seep out into your food. The same goes for drinking bottles; stick to glass or stainless steel bottles, both of which are BPA free. If you must drink from a plastic bottle, make sure that you do not leave the bottle in the car or exposed to bright sunlight, or the chemicals present in the bottles may seep into your drinking water.

Eating Out Like a Cavewoman

I travel and eat in restaurants a lot, and I don't find it difficult to stick to the Paleo Chic program. When possible, ask that your food be steamed, poached, or grilled without any sauce. Use lemon wedges, hot sauce, or mustard as condiments. Try to substitute a vegetable or salad instead of the potatoes or rice.

In a pinch, give the following options a whirl. Even if your options are not perfectly Paleo, they'll still be great choices because they're Paleo style. Don't beat yourself up if one meal isn't perfect. The rise in your cortisol levels just isn't worth the stress!

RESTAURANT OPTIONS

Vegetable omelet with a side of berries and a side of bacon
Steak and steamed broccoli with a large salad
Hamburger (no bun) with tomato and avocado slices
Grilled pork chop with sweet potato fries and a side salad
Grilled chicken over a salad
Grilled salmon and sautéed spinach
Seared lamb and asparagus
Beef carpaccio and steamed artichokes
Grilled chicken, plantains, guacamole, and salsa

Many restaurants now offer gluten-free menus, so don't be shy about asking! Also request that your food be cooked in olive oil or butter, and ask for olive oil and vinegar or lemon juice to dress your salad.

EATING ON THE ROAD OR IN THE SKIES: BYOF

Traveling with food might make you feel like a granny, but in reality you're treating yourself like an elite athlete, because that's exactly what they do. Restaurants along highways are usually fast-food places that offer nothing for cavewomen to eat. Airport food is superexpensive and supertasteless. If you're taking a road trip, pack a small cooler with Paleo-friendly foods—it's one less thing to worry about!

Flights are too often subject to delays and cancellations. Bringing your own food eliminates the stress and anxiety about how you're going to feed yourself when stuck in the middle of nowheresville. You'll arrive at your destination without any extra bloating from those salty, starchy foods served onboard. It's easy to say, "No, thank you," to a bag of chips when you are munching on some homemade trail mix.

Traveling with kids? Keeping your family well fed means no more temper tantrums due to hypoglycemia. If your child has food allergies, you're already well versed in how important it is to bring your own grub. There's enough to worry about when traveling these days; it's a relief not to have to worry about food.

Individual Packets of Whey or Goat Protein Powder. These are an absolute lifesaver for a snack or meal replacement! The protein provides satiety and will keep your energy levels balanced throughout the day. Measure out 1 to 2 scoops per portion, and ration out into individual Ziploc bags. Then dump into a shake bottle, add water, and voila! Instant satisfaction.

Powdered Green Drinks. Drinking green vegetable powders will detoxify the liver, boost energy, and provide valuable trace minerals to keep your blood sugar and mood stable. Pack your powders in a Ziploc and bring a shake bottle with you to help efficiently dissolve the powder in water.

Sardines in Olive Oil. Sardines are rich in essential fatty acids, so they'll keep your brain biochemistry balanced throughout the day. This means a happier you during the day and no chocolate cravings at night. You'll also get the benefits of a quality protein to maintain lean muscle mass even if you're forced to be strapped into a seat while traveling.

Vegetables. Cut up your favorite veggies. Wrap them in damp paper towels before placing them in a BPA-free container the night before your trip to keep them fresh for up to twelve hours. Vegetables are not only chock-full of antioxidants but also contain water to help keep you hydrated.

Nuts. Nature's ultimate fast food contain a powerful balance of protein, carbs, and fats. Measure out ¼-cup portions and place into individual containers. Crunch away your stress with almonds and cashews while getting the benefits of zinc, magnesium, balanced blood sugar, and neurotransmitter balance. If nuts are a trigger food for you, and you tend to overeat them, travel with limited amounts.

Jerky. This is a convenient way to get some quality proteins throughout your day. Look for pastured and grass-fed varieties so that you can also enjoy some omega-3s while feeding your inner cavewoman! Go to Steve's Paleogoods (www.stevesoriginal.com) for the best options, or make your own ahead of time.

Low-Glycemic Protein Bars. Protein bars are at the bottom of the list because they are a processed food full of sugars and poor-quality proteins. But in a pinch, they'll do the trick. Look for a gluten-free, whole-foods bar with whey protein as the primary fuel source, or make your own (see Recipes section, page 197).

Other Travel Nibbles. Hard-boiled eggs, canned wild Alaskan salmon, dried seaweed snacks, cherry tomatoes, carrots, plain Greek yogurt (full fat), apples, bananas, cooked shrimp, kale chips, homemade trail mix with nuts, seeds, chopped-up jerky pieces, and dried coconut.

CHAPTER 11

Paleo Supplements

One of the questions that people ask me most frequently is whether or not supplements are necessary. My answer is always yes! We live our lives at warp speed and put our bodies under far more stress than our ancestors ever did. Working long hours, constant exposure to technology, electromagnetic fields, and processed foods increase the nutritional demands on our bodies and tax our systems. On top of this, today's farmlands are deficient in trace minerals, leaving our fruits and vegetables with far less nutritional value than they had even two generations ago. Organic foods have significantly higher nutrient levels than commercially farmed foods, but bear in mind that even organic foods lose their nutrients if not eaten while fresh. If food has traveled across the country or from another continent, more nutrients will be lost. Get my point?

Before you pull out your hair in frustration, know that there's a lot you can do for yourself by eating clean, relaxing and enjoying your life, and taking supplements. Even I don't eat Paleo all the time; it's not always available to me, and I don't make myself crazy about it. I focus on the bigger picture, eat clean, drink plenty of water, and work at getting enough sleep and exercise. Don't sweat the small stuff. Fruits and vegetables are always better nutritional choices when compared with soda and processed foods. Every little healthy thing you do will have an impact. My diet is not perfect every day, and I often struggle to manage stress, so I take supplements every day. Just do the best you can; you'll still be making great changes for yourself!

KEEP IT FRESH

Just as you would do with your food, you need to make sure that your supplements are fresh and used within two years of production. The US Food and Drug Administration's Current Good Manufacturing Practice (cGMP) doesn't require expiration dates on dietary supplement product labels, but if one is used, it must be supported by stability testing data. However, as these regulations are still evolving, the FDA has yet to define what it considers to be adequate data. A quality supplement company will print the date of manufacture (the date the product in the bottle was produced) rather than an expiration date; in most cases, products are considered stable at full potency for two years from the manufacture date. Store your supplements in a cool, dry place, or refrigerate when necessary, for best stability and shelf life.

Why Take Supplements?

Why take supplements when eating a whole-foods diet? Let me tick off some great reasons:

1. Our farmlands are running seriously low in trace minerals and nutrients from overfarming, and our exposure to pollutants is through the roof. The environment is writing checks our bodies can't cash.
2. Life in the twenty-first century is stressful. Stress depletes

the vitamins and hormones in our bodies. We need to learn how to calm down and manage our stress better. Supplements, along with mind-body-spirit techniques, can be a supportive adjunct to lifestyle changes.

3. By the time our fruits and vegetables arrive at supermarkets, they have been trucked cross-country or flown in from other continents, which means that they are at least a week old—even if grown organically. Their nutrients start to dissipate as soon as they are harvested, so we need to supplement them with vitamins and minerals.

4. It's not what we eat, it's what we absorb. The nutrients in our foods are only as good as what our digestive tracts can assimilate. Digestive enzymes are a must for 95 percent of people out there, unless you're one of the lucky few with a fully functioning intestinal tract. If you've ever taken just one dose of antibiotics, you know how they can alter your body's ability to produce digestive enzymes properly. Nutrients are lost during food processing and handling. Yes, you may be buying organic olive oil, but it may still be lower in vitamin E content than if you were able to buy it fresh-pressed due to how it was processed and handled.

5. If you're eating meat that isn't grass fed or fish that isn't wild, you may be exposing yourself to antibiotics and hormones fed to animals. Antibiotics can wipe out the good intestinal bacteria, making it difficult for B vitamins to be absorbed through the intestinal walls.

6. We all know that sunscreen is important in the fight against skin cancer. But using sunscreen and staying out of the sun means that many of us are now deficient in vitamin D_3. Even my clients in Florida require supplementation. If you can't take a thirty-minute walk in the sunshine every day, then take 10,000 IU (international units) of D_3 every other day until your blood levels of D_3 reach 80 ng/dL (nanograms per deciliter of blood). Then take 5,000 IU a

day for maintenance. Make sure that you get a blood test twice a year to check your vitamin D_3 levels.

7. Birth control pills increase the need for probiotics, B_6, vitamin C, zinc, and riboflavin (B_2). If you're not getting enough of these from your diet, then supplements are essential.

8. Exercise, although beneficial, increases our nutritional requirements for muscle repair and growth. It is next to impossible to recover from a strenuous workout and prevent injuries without proper nutrition.

Before Getting Started . . .

The following protocols will help you heal your body and get your metabolism stoked once again. These protocols are based on my eighteen years of experience treating clients, clinical research, and case studies from some of the best practitioners in the field. Some girls want designer jeans; I just want designer supplements!

The suggestions in this chapter are natural-remedy guidelines. Check with your nutritionally oriented physician, nutritionist, or other medical practitioner before taking any supplements.

You don't have to take all of the supplements suggested if you'd rather not. Introduce one at a time to see if there is any change in how you feel. Small, consistent changes can make a big difference. Which brings me to my next point: the supplements always work better in your body than in the bottle, so remember to take them regularly. Buy yourself a pretty pillbox that you can keep in your handbag so they'll always be handy. And take them as directed.

Last but not least, know that a fistful of vitamins alone won't keep you healthy; joy and laughter are the greatest nutrients of all. They can feed your soul and nourish your spirit! Health plus a negative mind-set equals baditude; health plus a positive outlook equals gratitude!

Unless specified otherwise, all supplements should be taken with food. Make sure that each of your meals contains some fat to help your body absorb fat-soluble vitamins A, D, E, and K. Supplements are listed under each health concern in order of their importance and effectiveness.

Basic Foundation Protocol

Prebiotics, also called fermentable fiber, are indigestible food ingredients that feed probiotics and help them grow. They can be found most commonly in supplement form as FOS (fructooligosaccharides). Probiotics are healthy bacteria that populate the gastrointestinal tract. They are responsible for a healthy gut and immune system and facilitate digestion and detoxification. Prebiotics and probiotics are generally found in fermented dairy products, but those are not necessarily part of a cavewoman's diet. The Paleo diet includes more protein than other regimens, increasing the need for other sources of probiotics. What's a cavewoman to do?

- Eat foods rich in prebiotics such as Jerusalem artichokes, dandelion greens, garlic, leeks, onions, and bananas.
- Stick to the Paleo diet and eat a variety of fresh vegetables, including kale, chard, spinach, broccoli, cauliflower, and any others rich in soluble, prebiotic fiber.
- Purchase medical-grade prebiotics and probiotics. Most health food stores sell strains that are dead because the probiotics are not shipped and stored properly. I recommend purchasing your supplements through a holistic health care practitioner, as they typically have quality products manufactured to a higher standard. For natural sources of probiotics, eat fermented foods such as pickles and

sauerkraut. If you can tolerate dairy, drink raw milk and the fermented form known as kefir.

- Stress management is the foundation of good gut health. Stress depletes stomach acid and flattens out the delicate walls of the GI tract, leading to food allergies and a leaky gut (intestinal hyperpermeability). Incorporate at least ten minutes of deep breathing into your day (bedtime is always my fave time to unwind) and take a yoga class twice a week. Exercise at least three to four times a week and do one thing every day that makes your heart sing, like blasting your favorite music, dancing around the house, calling a good friend, or spending quality time with family or friends.
- Also noteworthy is that all detoxification reactions in the body are vitamin D_3 dependent; that is why it's included in this protocol.

SUPPLEMENTS

Probiotics	50 billion 2 times a day.
Digestive enzymes	As needed with the HCl acid test. (See box on opposite page.)
Vitamin D_3	10,000 IU (international units) every other day until your blood levels of D_3 reach 80 ng/dL (nanograms per deciliter). Then 5,000 IU a day for maintenance.
Omega-3	2 to 3 teaspoons of liquid omega-3s a day (this is equivalent to 2,000-3,000 mg per day).

Magnesium	10 mg/kg (milligrams per kilogram). (This equals about 1,000 mg a day.) Once your values reach 6.8 in an RBC (red blood cell) magnesium blood test, you can lower your dosage accordingly.
Zinc	25 mg to 50 mg a day; increase your dosage until you reach 1,400 mcg/dL in a RBC zinc blood test.
Curcumin	1,400-mg capsule a day.

TESTING, TESTING, ONE, TWO, THREE

Your intestinal tract requires the production of stomach acids to break down food. Stomach acid contains hydrochloric acid (HCl), potassium chloride, and sodium chloride. Most people don't produce sufficient HCl to break down food properly, as evidenced by the pharmaceutical products out there to treat gas, reflux, belching, and heartburn—which are usually caused by a deficiency in HCl! If you are low in HCl, not only won't you absorb nutrients from food, but also you'll put yourself at risk for deficiencies of trace minerals and B vitamins, as well as lose calcium, vitamin C, and beta-carotene.

Contrary to popular belief, reflux and heartburn in adults are caused most often by *low* stomach acid. As we age, our body produces less and less HCl. The lower esophageal sphincter, a ring of muscle at the junction of the esophagus and the stomach, is actually held closed by adequate HCl. If HCl is low, the sphincter creeps open, allowing the stomach acid to splash upward. Antacids are a quick fix, but they can have long-term side effects such as bone loss and anemia and will never cure the problem.

The ultimate goal is to replenish HCl stores so that the sphincter stays closed.

To test your stomach acid, purchase a bottle of 200-milligram betaine HCl capsules. (*Caution: Do not perform this test if you have peptic ulcers.* Rather, consult a nutritionally oriented physician for treatment.)

In the middle of your next solid meal, take one 200-milligram capsule of HCl. Wait thirty minutes and see if you feel any mild burning in your stomach. At each subsequent meal, increase the HCl dose by one capsule: one at breakfast, two at lunch, three at dinner, and so forth, until you feel the mild burning. If you feel a burning at four capsules, for example, subtract one capsule and take three at every meal. To relieve the burning, drink a large glass of water to dilute the acid.

Do not take more than seven capsules during the HCl test. If you take seven and feel nothing, it means that you are severely deficient in HCl. If so, pick up a bottle of 500-milligram betaine HCl capsules, and repeat the test, starting at 1 capsule per meal. If you get to 3 and nothing happens, *do not exceed 1,500 milligrams.* This is the maximum amount you should take at one meal. If you take more than this amount, your body will not learn to make HCl on its own—which is ultimately the goal.

If you notice that you take 3 capsules per meal for a few months, and the burning sensation reappears, then you can decrease the dose to 2 capsules per meal. Taper down and repeat as necessary until you get to your maintenance dose (or none at all). And if you are stressed out, you may need to temporarily increase your HCl dosage, as stress can make you stop producing stomach acid. Add some yoga or meditation to your routine to reestablish balance.

Cortisol Control

The hormone cortisol is a low-grade form of adrenaline. Cortisol is your conditional friend because it has anabolic potential, which means that it can help your body build muscle. You want to get your cortisol level up during your workouts, but the rest of the time, you need to keep that baby in line! Since so much of cortisol production is linked to lifestyle and stress management, try to unwind and let go of the day's stress *before* you climb into bed at night. Here's how to be the mistress of your cortisol:

- Eat breakfast within an hour of waking up, eat at regular intervals throughout the day, and don't skip meals.

- Control your carb intake. Too many carbs can jack up your insulin level, which, in turn, signals your body to release cortisol into the bloodstream.

- Maintain good sleep habits with nightly rituals such as reading, deep breathing, stretching, or meditating. Lights must be out no later than eleven o'clock; ideally by ten. Aim for a minimum of seven to eight hours of sleep each night.

- Drink coffee thirty minutes to an hour before working out. If you need some caffeine throughout the day, drink green tea, which contains L-theanine. This calming amino acid can positively impact the brainwaves that promote relaxation.

- Limit your heavy lifting workouts to sixty minutes (unless you are walking or doing yoga) and your high-intensity interval training to thirty minutes. Longer workouts can raise and keep your cortisol levels elevated for hours after you finish, resulting in fitful sleep. Here comes that three-in-the-morning wakeup call!

SUPPLEMENTS

Licorice root, 7:1 extract	500 mg (milligrams) first thing in the morning on an empty stomach.
Rhodiola rosea	200 mg 2 times a day.
Holy basil	600 mg a day.
Inositol powder	3,000 mg to 6,000 mg a day.
Phosphatidylserine	400 mg at bedtime.

Detoxification

Liver Detox

This is a great protocol to clean out the toxic wasteland in your body via your liver. If you feel sluggish in spite of good sleep, have dark brown circles under your eyes, PMS, joint pains, or wake up between the hours of one and three nightly, then this liver cleansing is for you. These symptoms are signs that your liver is having a hard time trying to detoxify itself. Poor liver function also means that you may have a hard time detoxifying estrogen and cortisol.

- Be sure to drink a glass of freshly juiced greens once a day or drink 1 tablespoon of PaleoGreens mixed with 8 ounces of water three times a day.

- Saunas are the it-girl of beauty treatments and detoxification. Infrared saunas can pull out toxins such as metals and plastics, while heat saunas can facilitate fat loss. To get rid of those toxins and stay hydrated, drink ice water in a metal bottle while basking in the glow of the sauna's dry heat. Try to hit the hot box for fifteen minutes at least three times per week.

SUPPLEMENTS

Forty-five minutes before a sauna treatment, take the following:

Vitamin C	2,000 mg (milligrams).
Vitamin E	400 IU (international units).
R-alpha lipoic acid	300 mg.
Spanish black radish	750 mg 3 times a day for 2 months; then reduce to 1,100 mg.
Milk thistle	150 mg 2 times.
Globe artichoke leaf	400 mg 2 times.
Dandelion root	200 mg 2 times.
N-acetyl cysteine (NAC)	1,000 mg.

Heavy Metal Detox

Although heavy metals occur naturally in nature, they can be harmful to the body in large quantities. Trace amounts of heavy metals such as mercury, cadmium, and lead enter the body from food, water, and air. Our bodies store these metals in tissues such as the brain, kidneys, intestines, and fat. Over time, and with continual exposure, heavy metals can build to the point of toxicity. High levels of heavy metals in the body can cause symptoms such as fatigue, insomnia, hypothyroidism, weight gain, yeast and sinus infections, and irritable bowel syndrome. So detoxing them will be imperative for getting your health back.

The protocol listed above provides guidelines that you should follow in your treatment, but *only* when working with a nutritionally oriented practitioner. You will need to be supervised throughout your detoxification process. Everyone reacts differently to detoxification, so go about it carefully—it's your body and your health.

The DMPS (dimercaptopropane sulfonic acid) challenge is the most reliable way to test your body's levels of heavy metals. DMPS is a chelating agent that will pull mercury out of the body as efficiently as possible. DMSA (dimercaptosuccinic acid) is an oral chelating agent that can displace mercury and expose it to the brain, so unless you know your genetic profile or are working with a qualified practitioner, don't mess with it. Heavy metals are stubborn suckers. You have to find a good practitioner to mobilize the metals from their storage sites and eliminate them from the body. And you need to protect your brain and internal organs from metals as they leave your body.

Visit the American College for Advancement in Medicine (www .acam.org) to find a nutritionally oriented MD in your area who can do the testing for you, and give you chelation and nutritional therapy if needed. Once you have metals, you will need to manage them for a lifetime. Even if you carefully avoid mercury-laden fish, remove your mercury-based dental fillings, and keep a green home, the environment is a constant source of pollutants.

As you go through your detox, hop into an infrared sauna for fifteen minutes at least three times a week to help flush toxins from the blood and eliminate them via the sweat glands.

- Dissolve two cups Epsom salts in a warm bath and soak for twenty minutes.
- Exercise is a great detoxifier too!
- Make sure that your diet is rich in protein and fiber to support detoxification in both the liver and the gut, where metals love to hang out.
- PectaSol, which is a form of modified citrus pectin, helps clear out mercury from the microvilli of the intestines. (Dosage listed below.)
- Sprinkle two tablespoons of flax meal or chia seeds into your salads or smoothies to give you a daily dose of fiber.

SUPPLEMENTS

PectaSol	3 capsules 2 times a day, 30 minutes before meals for active detox; 1 capsule 2 times a day, 30 minutes before meals for maintenance.
Chlorophyll complex	10 capsules a day.
R-alpha lipoic acid	300 mg (milligrams) a day.
Vitamin C	2,000 mg 3 times a day.
Aqueous selenium	600 mcg (micrograms) a day.

Probiotics	75 billion a day.
Magnesium	400 mg 2 times a day.
Vitamin B complex	50 mg a day.
Omega-3	1 tablespoon a day (3,000 mg-liquid form).
Multivitamin with trace minerals	As directed.

Sugar Detox

Because of the addictive effects that sugar has on brain biochemistry, your body can experience withdrawal symptoms when you give it up. Ease these symptoms by following the Paleo Chic program and eating plenty of fats, protein, and dark green leafy veggies. Every time you want to reach for chocolate, grab half an avocado and some shredded chicken or raw nuts and seeds instead to nip those cravings in the bud. Avoid diet sodas and artificial sweeteners and use stevia instead, and quell cravings with 1 tablespoon organic cocoa powder and ⅛ teaspoon stevia steeped in 8 ounces of boiling water. Once your taste buds adjust to low-sugar living, the sweet stuff won't taste so good anymore.

Any time you have a food craving, mix 5 to 10 grams of glutamine powder in 1 tablespoon of heavy cream and drink it. You'll be amazed how quickly it works! L-glutamine is an amino acid that is essential for the health of the immune system and digestive tract. It strengthens the mucosal cells and in turn helps leaky gut and sugar cravings. Glutamine also helps promote optimal muscle growth and strength and has shown to be particularly useful in helping prevent muscle wasting.

Supplements

Gymnema leaf, 10:1 extract	400 mg (milligram) twice a day.
Chromium nicotinate glycinate chelate	300 mcg (micrograms) 3 times a day.
Taurine	500 mg 3 times a day.
Vanadium nicotinate glycinate chelate	100 mcg 3 times a day.
Omega-3	1 tablespoon a day (3,000 mg-liquid form).

Estrogen Cleanse

How do you know if your body is circulating excess estrogens? If you have PMS, irregular and/or heavy bleeding during your monthly period, migraines, polycystic ovarian syndrome, insulin resistance, endometriosis, fibroids, ovarian cysts, and/or breast cancer, you are very likely circulating excess estrogens that are not excreted by the body. You can also get your blood levels checked through a nutritionally oriented physician to monitor your estrogen-to-progesterone ratio.

- Maintain intestinal health and bowel regularity by eating 30 grams of dietary fiber every day. The fiber found in flax meal can bind to estrogen so that it will be readily excreted from the body. Add 2 tablespoons of flax meal to smoothies, juices, or applesauce.

- Reduce exposure to plastics.

- Avoid gluten.

- Drink plenty of freshly juiced greens and eat liver-supporting foods such as Brussels sprouts, broccoli, cauliflower, artichokes, dandelion greens, radishes, and beets.

- Eat lots of dark leafy greens to support liver function and provide you with extra lignans that will bind to estrogen and help the body excrete it.

- If you drink alcoholic beverages, make it red wine. Even moderate alcohol consumption increases estrogen levels in both men and women. Red wine that is rich in resveratrol has been shown to lower estrogen levels. Aim for no more than a glass of red wine once or twice a week. Sardinian and Spanish wines make good choices, as do Pinot Noirs and Merlots.

- Get adequate exercise and control your weight to curtail the overproduction of estrogen. Excess body fat results in conservation of estrogen, but lowering your body fat can reduce your hormonal burden.

SUPPLEMENTS

Omega-3	1 tablespoon a day (3,000 mg-liquid form).
Vitamin B complex	50 mg (milligrams) a day.
Diindolylmethane (DIM)	200 mg 2 times a day for 2 months; then 200 mg a day maintenance.
Calcium D-glucarate	1,500 mg a day.

Taurine	1,000 mg a day.
Milk thistle	300 mg a day with breakfast.
Flax meal	2 tablespoons a day.

Exercise

When it comes to working out, there are steps you can take before and after you exercise to light a fire under those fat-burning hormones:

Preworkout

Put the right balance of nutrients into your body before a workout to improve energy use and insulin sensitivity. You can exercise on an empty stomach if you prefer, but I recommend eating protein and fats at least one hour before activity to boost your brain neurotransmitters and optimize your performance. Limit your fructose intake so that you can access and mobilize your body fat stores during your workout. Pears, melons, berries, figs, dates, pineapple, apples, and raisins are all high in fructose, so save them for your postworkout meal.

SUPPLEMENTS

Take one hour before your workout.

L-carnitine	3,000 mg (milligrams).
Omega-3	1 tablespoon (3,000 mg-liquid form).

| Branched-chain amino acids (BCAAs) | 10 g (grams). |
| Caffeine | 1 cup coffee or tea. |

Postworkout

Take the supplements listed below, along with a postworkout shake, within ten minutes of finishing your workout. This will help your body repair and build muscle tissue, increase free testosterone, and lower your cortisol levels. Cortisol inhibits the release of growth hormone, so if you want to build those gorgeous muscles, then clearing your cortisol with a postworkout shake is a must.

SUPPLEMENTS

Vitamin C	2,000 mg.
Branched-chain amino acids (BCAAs)	10 g.
Magnesium	600 mg.
Glutamine powder	10 g in powdered form, dissolved in water.
Vitamin E	400 IU (international units).
Phosphatidylserine	400 mg at bedtime.

POSTWORKOUT MUSCLE MOCKTAIL

I recommend making your shake at home and taking it with you to the gym so that you can enjoy it immediately following your workout.

1 to 2 scoops whey protein powder.

1 cup unsweetened almond milk, coconut milk, coconut water, or water.

1 cup frozen or fresh fruit, such as berries, ½ banana, mangoes, and so on.

Cinnamon

Blend with ice and a dash of cinnamon; the ice will keep it fresh until ready for consumption.

Fat Burning

- Sleep is both a fat-loss and an anabolic nutrient, so make sure you hit the hay by ten o'clock and get at least seven to eight hours of sleep, or more if your body requires it.
- Eat plenty of protein, fiber, and quality fats at each meal to help your body access its own fat stores.
- Avoid sugar, artificial sweeteners, and excess booze, which will not only spread your waistline but also hit the pause button on your fat-burning efforts.
- Do a combination of high-intensity interval training and lifting heavy weights at the gym at least four times a week to give you rapid results in the least amount of time. Work it!

Supplements

Branched-chain amino acids (BCAAs)	10 g (grams) preworkout and postworkout.
L-carnitine	3,000 mg (milligrams) preworkout.
Omega-3	1 tablespoon (liquid form) preworkout.
Coenzyme Q	200 mg preworkout.
Probiotics	50 billion a day.
Zinc	25 mg to 50 mg a day.
Organic coconut oil	1 tablespoon a day.

Muscle Recovery

Flooding your cells with protein and antioxidants after a workout will help lower high cortisol levels generated during activity and enable the muscle tissue to begin repairing itself immediately. This postworkout shake will also reduce delayed onset muscle soreness.

Within ten minutes of finishing your workout, make yourself the following shake:

POSTWORKOUT REPLETION SHAKE

1 heaping tablespoon of
glutamine powder
1 to 2 scoops of protein
powder
1 cup berries
1 scoop of greens powder

1 cup coconut milk or
coconut water
½ cup water
1 teaspoon cinnamon
⅛ teaspoon stevia powder
to sweeten

Combine all ingredients in blender with a handful of ice cubes until thoroughly mixed.

SUPPLEMENTS

Magnesium	See box on the following page for daily dosage.
Branched-chain amino acids (BCAAs)	10 g (grams) preworkout and postworkout.
Coconut water	8 ounces postworkout.
Topical magnesium	Apply 2 pumps behind your knees at bedtime.

MAGNIFICENT MAGNESIUM!

World-renowned strength and nutrition coach Charles Poliquin really hammered home for me the message about how critical the mineral magnesium is to our health. Magnesium, a nutritional superstar, is responsible for more than three hundred chemical reactions in the human body and the baseline energetics of all cells. It's one of the most abundant minerals in our body, with most of it stored in bones, which is why insufficient magnesium leads to osteopenia and osteoporosis.

Magnesium affects all of our hormones. It helps maintain our insulin level. Our muscles depend on magnesium, too; when I worked in hospital cardiac units, heart attack patients were always given a hefty dose to relax the cardiac muscle. Magnesium relaxes skeletal muscle, making it an important part of your postworkout nutrition requirements. You also need magnesium to detoxify and control the stress hormone cortisol following a workout.

We are grossly deficient in this mineral because our farmlands have been depleted with overuse and contain almost none. Even if you can scrounge up some magnesium-rich soil, most commercial fertilizers actually block the absorption of minerals by plants. We are also chugging sugar-rich sodas that are high in phosphorous and provoke the body to excrete magnesium. Stress causes the body to dump magnesium, too.

When combined with exercise, magnesium can boost testosterone and DHEA levels, and improve muscle mass gains and insulin sensitivity.

Want to know your magnesium levels? You can measure them with a red blood cell magnesium blood test. (You can order the test online at LEF.org.) The closer you are to the optimal level of 6.8, the greater your general health will be. You will improve your blood glucose, cortisol, blood pressure, and heart rhythms. The more optimal the magnesium levels in your tissues, the less you'll experience the adverse effects of stress. Take small dosages orally throughout the day, and use topical magnesium behind the knees or on the inside of your elbow at night to rock out your sleep.

Daily dosage: 10 mg/kg (milligrams per kilogram) for women, and 15 mg/kg to 20 mg/kg for men for twelve weeks. (This equals about 1,000 mg per day for women, and 2,000 mg per day for men.) Once your values reach 6.8 in an RBC magnesium test, you can lower your dosage accordingly. I suggest using a mixture of magnesiums (taurate, orotate, glycinate, and fumarate) to avoid stomach upset and get the most absorption bang for your buck.

Gut Healing

This is a great protocol for treating heartburn, leaky gut syndrome, food allergies, autoimmune conditions, *Helicobacter pylori* (the bacterium responsible for most ulcers) and ulcers, irritable bowel syndrome, weaning yourself off proton pump inhibitors (PPIs, a class of drugs used to suppress stomach acid production), and reestablishing the normal gut flora (especially after a round of antibiotics).

- Follow the cavewoman diet to speed up healing, since protein rebuilds the walls of your digestive system.

- Avoid food allergens, gluten, and sugars, since they irritate the gut and promote inflammation.

- Drink chamomile and slippery elm tea to soothe the GI tract.

- Toss some okra in a soup or stew; the slippery, slimy insides of the vegetable act as a demulcent to coat and soothe the stomach.

- Grind up fresh flaxseeds (flax meal) or chia seeds and add 1 to 2 tablespoons to salads, smoothies, or applesauce to get the demulcent benefits.

- Drink green juices to promote healing from within. Their nutrients are in their raw state and contain many biologically active enzymes to put your system back in balance. When fiber and pulp are removed, nutrients can be passively absorbed across the gut wall, requiring little to no work from your digestive tract. If you have a Vitamix blender, blend up whole green vegetables—spinach, kale, cabbage, Swiss chard, you name it—to get the added benefits of fiber from vegetables. If you're on the go, belly up to the juice bar for a shot of wheatgrass or other green drink, and get on with your day. To keep it uber simple, toss a heaping tablespoon of powdered greens in a tall cup of H_2O on the rocks, cover, and give it a few good shakes before drinking.

Give this cocktail a whirl:

GORGEOUSLY GREEN

2 stalks celery	1 Swiss chard leaf
½ cucumber	Bunch fresh cilantro or
½ apple	parsley
½ lemon	5 kale leaves
½ lime	Handful of spinach leaves
½-inch piece peeled ginger	

When making juices, wash all vegetables and fruits before using, buy organic produce whenever possible, and peel or slice off the lemon rind and the white pith. Also, to juice small leaves such as parsley and cilantro, roll them up into a ball to compact the leaves.

SUPPLEMENTS

Glutamine powder	1 tablespoon mixed in 8 ounces water 4 times a day.
Probiotics	25 billion 3 times a day.
Deglycyrrhizinated licorice (DGL)	Chew four 400 mg (milligram) tablets between meals for acute symptoms; maintenance dose is 1 to 2 tablets 20 minutes before meals.
Omega-3	1 teaspoon (1,000 mg liquid form) 3 times a day.
Zinc carnosine	75 mg 2 times a day.

Belly 911

Do you have digestive woes from too much partying last night or going off your cavewoman diet? When tummy troubles strike, I reach for three ingredients: fresh ginger, mint, and fennel. For a stomach-soothing herbal tea, steep 1 teaspoon of each in hot water with some orange zest for three to five minutes; strain and drink immediately.

Digest Ease

For a morning-after food hangover or booze cleanse, toss the following in a juicer for some blessed relief:

FANTASTICALLY FRESH

½ cucumber	2 mint sprigs, rolled up
1 green apple	¼-inch to ½-inch piece of
1 stalk fennel with leaves	ginger

Put all ingredients in a juicer. Pour into a tall glass and enjoy.

REPRODUCTIVE HORMONE BALANCING

- Amp up your protein and dark greens to punch through hormonal distress—especially during the second half of your monthly cycle.

- Yoga twice per week can also help level out your hormones.

- Chaste tree is an herb that does an incredible job at balancing the endocrine system and supporting normal progesterone levels. Time and again, I have helped women reestablish ovulation and normal cycles when taking chaste tree, especially for those who are amenorrheic or transitioning off oral contraceptives. (*Never* take chaste tree if you're taking oral contraceptives). If you have strong menstrual cramps, breast tenderness, bloating, or hot flashes, then chaste tree may be right for you. If, however, you have minor menstrual cramps, then this is a likely sign that you are already progesterone dominant, so chaste tree would be contraindicated.

This is a great vitamin cocktail for getting your hormonal groove back. If you need to restore your menses, have PMS, are going through menopause, or just feel off-kilter, then give this regimen a try.

SUPPLEMENTS

Vitamin D_3	5,000 IU (international units) a day; more if your vitamin D_3 level is below 60 ng/dL (nanograms per deciliter of blood).
Diindolylmethane (DIM)	200 mg (milligrams) a day.
Chaste tree, 6:1 extract from Vitex agnus-castus fruit	500 mg first thing in the morning.
Omega-3	1 tablespoon a day (approximately 3,000 mg of omega-3s).
Primrose oil	1,000 mg gel cap 2 times a day.

Stress Management

The following protocol will help lower your cortisol, promote restful sleep, and keep your energy grooving evenly throughout the day:

- Eating clean can make or break you when it comes to handling stress. Think about how your body feels when it runs on coffee and bagels versus a vegetable omelet and fresh fruit. Some foods (carbs) can overstimulate you, while others (protein) can help you remain calm and clear.

- Give your body plenty of TLC if you're stressed: eat regularly, drink chamomile tea, be consistent with your workouts, take hot baths, and get some quiet downtime each and every day. We may not be able to control all the stress that comes our way, but we can certainly handle how we react to it.

- Taurine is a depressant that calms down the brain.

- Taking vitamin C immediately following a workout lowers cortisol and boosts testosterone.

SUPPLEMENTS

Omega-3	2,000 mg (liquid or capsule form) a day with food, preferably before working out.
Magnesium	Start with 400 mg 2 times a day; increase as needed.
Rhodiola rosea	200 mg 2 times a day.
Phosphatidylserine	400 mg a day at bedtime.
Vitamin C	2,000 mg immediately after workout.
Taurine	1,000 mg a day.

Sleep Restoration

Sleep recovery is a complex issue because the root causes can be many. There are different approaches you can take to get a better night's sleep.

Balance Blood Sugar

If you wake up around one in the morning, it may be due to a stress hormone response fueled by hypoglycemia. The best solution is to eat a snack closer to bedtime with the right mix of proteins and fiber-rich carbohydrates to help you sleep deeply and for longer amounts of time. Think chicken salad and tomatoes, salmon and broccoli, or turkey with broccoli. I'm talking one or two bites' worth here—nothing extravagant. A teaspoon of almond or cashew butter might do the trick. Experiment and see what works best for you.

Boosting Neurotransmitters

A great way to boost your brain neurotransmitters and get your brain happy and craving-free is to eat meat and nuts at every meal, and to make sure that your gut is healthy. Your gut plays a huge role in your sleeping well at night. Most people think that serotonin is produced in the brain, but it's actually produced in your gut. If you have internal inflammation such as colitis or Crohn's disease, diarrhea, or overuse of antibiotics, insomnia and depression can develop as a result. Your gut rules your brain, so treat it kindly. And if you are taking gamma-aminobutyric acid (GABA) and not sleeping or feeling better, you probably have some intestinal issues, such as food allergies or intolerances that you need to address. (See the "Gut Healing" section for more information.)

Magnesium

The more magnesium you have in your tissues, the less your body will overreact to stress. When you are stressed out, your body makes norepinephrine—a hormone that functions like a neurotransmitter and gets released during the body's fight-or-flight response. But if you take optimal amounts of magnesium, you will

mitigate the catecholamine response, and improve both the quality
and the quantity of your sleep.

SUPPLEMENTS

Magnesium glycinate	400 mg (milligrams) before bed.
Topical magnesium	Evenly distribute 1 to 2 pumps of topical magnesium behind the knees or inside the elbows. The skin is thinner here, and the cream will be better absorbed.
Gamma-aminobutyric acid (GABA)	200 mg to 400 mg at bedtime.

Exercise-Induced Insomnia

If you are overtraining and waking up at three in the morning,
lower your cortisol with the following nutrients.

SUPPLEMENTS

Vitamin C	2,000 mg (milligrams) immediately after workout or with breakfast.
Phosphatidylserine	400 mg immediately after workout or with dinner.
Rhodiola rosea	200 mg 2 times a day.
Vitamin B$_6$	50 mg a day.

| Magnesium | 1200–2000 mg per day, or as tolerated. |
| Topical magnesium | Evenly distribute 1 to 2 pumps of topical magnesium behind the knees or inside the elbows. |

Anxiety-Induced Insomnia

Since sleep rules our metabolic kingdoms, we have to think about the impact of our lifestyle choices. What's the antidote to all of this? Think like a cavewoman. Unplug by nine o'clock at night. Get in a dark room. Clear out all external stimuli and technology. Eliminate toxins from your diet and your body. Relax. Breathe. Nighty night!

- Eat within one hour of waking up and at regular intervals throughout the day.

- Snack on 2 ounces sliced turkey breast one hour before bedtime to offset low blood sugar and boost serotonin levels in the brain.

- Have a small piece of fruit with five almonds before bed to boost serotonin levels.

- Cognitive behavioral therapy is an essential part of addressing anxiety and rewiring the brain; it helps to break the vicious cycle of repetitive thoughts and behaviors. Seek out a practitioner. Meditation is also a helpful activity (see CD mentioned on p. 190).

- Drink Yogi Bedtime Tea throughout the day if your anxiety is severe and steep up to 3 bags at one time; otherwise drink

1 cup with dinner or before bed while soaking in an Epsom salts bath.

- Get the alpha waves in your brain grooving with some meditation; deep breathing is remarkably effective at lowering cortisol. One of my favorite meditation CDs is *A Meditation to Help You with Healthful Sleep* by Belleruth Naparstek, available at Health Journeys (www .healthjourneys.com).

Supplements

Try taking the following combination of nutrients when anxiety strikes throughout the day or an hour before bedtime:

Holy basil	600 mg (milligrams).
Inositol powder	3,000 mg to 6,000 mg.
CatecholaCalm by Designs for Health	3 capsules up to 2 times a day (www.designsforhealth.com).
Magnesium glycinate	400 mg up to 3 times a day.
5-Hydroxytryptophan (5-HTP)	200 mg a day.
Taurine	1,000 mg 2 times a day.

BLOOD TESTS TO HAVE DONE

How many times have you had blood tests done at your annual physical by your primary care physician, only to hear that "everything looks normal"? What we need to understand is that today's medical model is based on the blood work of Homer Simpson: someone who is overweight with elevated insulin, cortisol, blood lipids, and a bad junk-food habit. So if you're healthier than Homer Simpson, you're going to just slip under the radar and fall through the cracks. It's all relative, isn't it?

If you are already working with a functional medicine doctor, he or she will determine which tests are right for you. My friend and colleague Dr. Mark Houston, Director of the Hypertension Institute of Nashville, and I composed the following list of tests that will give you the best picture of your overall health and get to the root of any chronic issues you've been having.

- Fasting insulin and/or glucose test. If results are abnormal, follow up with a glucose tolerance test (GTT): monitors insulin resistance

- SpectraCell micronutrient testing and Lipoprotein particle profile: measures vitamin, mineral, and antioxidant deficiencies and those at risk for coronary artery disease

- Triglycerides: measures fats in the blood

- C-reactive protein: measures level of systemic inflammation

- Lipoprotein (a): identifies risk of coronary artery disease

- Vitamin B_{12}: helps diagnose central nervous system disorders, anemia, malabsorption syndrome, fatigue

- Homocysteine: determines risk of arterial plaque formation

- Thyroid-stimulating hormone (TSH): first-line screening for thyroid disease; stimulates the thyroid to produce T_3 and T_4

- Triiodothyronine (T_3): determines the active form of thyroid hormone present

- Thyroxine, Free (Free T_4): a more sensitive test for thyroid hormone production

- Reverse T_3: tests thyroid resistance and the body's ability to convert T_4 to T_3

- 25-hydroxy vitamin D: important to every cell and tissue in the body

- Gluten antibodies: helps diagnose or monitor celiac disease

- Estradiol (E_2): helps evaluate hormonal imbalances

- Testosterone (total and free): the principal anabolic steroid directing metabolism and the repair and regeneration of healthy tissues

- LEAP mediator release test (MRT): tests for allergies in 130 foods and 20 chemicals and additives

- Heavy metals panel: tests for the presence of heavy metals in the body

- RBC zinc: assesses intracellular zinc status

- RBC magnesium: assesses intracellular magnesium status

- Urinalysis and microalbumin: tests for diabetes, urinary tract infections, and kidney disease

- Iron and total iron-binding capacity (TIBC): tests for iron-deficiency anemia

- Comprehensive metabolic panel (CMP): evaluates the functioning of the body's major organs, such as the heart, liver, kidneys, glands, nerves, bones, and muscles

Conclusion

Paleo Chic is an ultramodern approach to an ancient idea. It's about getting back to our roots, detoxing, reestablishing balance, and giving ourselves a metabolic makeover that keeps us moving forward. Every now and then, we forward-thinking women have to turbocharge our health. When we let that inner party girl dominate our health dojo for too long, we need to hit the reset button and get back on track.

It's so easy to get caught up in the whirlwind of Life 2.0 and neglect our primal needs. Modern living has so much to offer, but, now more than ever, it's important that we take the time to unplug and recharge ourselves. There are times when we need to take a break, turn off our phones, put down our iPads, and dial into our bodies' natural needs. Diets don't have to be as restrictive as a corset or as oppressive as a glass ceiling. A diet can actually make you feel your best and free you from all of the overbearing toxins, sugar, and food allergens that modern living can throw at even the most powerful women. Each of us has primal physical potential just waiting to be unleashed.

Paleo Chic isn't a one-size-fits-all diet of extreme clean all of the time. Being a gorgeous modern woman means striking a balance between what you enjoy and what you need. Finding that balance is different for all of us. Here's mine: I will always eat chocolate and drink martinis, but I will treat them as indulgences. And a big, sexy salad with piles of farm-fresh vegetables and some grilled steak or salmon and a hard-core workout totally turn me on. The challenge lies in figuring out what works for you and your body—and making peace with it.

Perhaps a Paleo-style breakfast of steak and avocado slices in place of a bowl of cereal and milk gives you the energy to close a big deal. Maybe you'll satisfy those afternoon cravings with a protein shake or a square of dark chocolate instead of a cupcake. Or maybe you'll want to go straight for the gold on the fourteen-day Paleo Detox that gets your year started with a bang. No matter which path you choose on your amazing journey, this Paleo Chic diet will reward you with remarkable changes in your body, mind, and spirit.

Paleo diets can be extreme, but Paleo Chic is not. Reaching goals requires tenacity, consistency, and a can-do attitude, but there will be times when life goes askew and your eating habits will too. That's okay. Both you and how you eat are what I like to call perfectly imperfect. Whatever happens, cut yourself some slack and respect the path of your personal evolution. Trust in your awareness and mindfulness to get you back on track. Even if you make mistakes and fall flat on your face, you're still moving forward, ultimately.

When I fall off the Paleo pony, it is usually because I haven't budgeted the time to pay attention to myself. I am sure you lead a full life and as a result will have to work at putting yourself first too. Think about what will get you motivated to go to the gym, turn down that office cake, and get yourself some sleep. Cavewomen didn't have half the responsibilities we have, and making time for yourself is half the battle.

So use this Paleo Chic diet well. Use it to drop the pounds in a jiffy, but also use it to feel empowered in your own skin and in your own life!

Live gorgeously,
Esther

Paleo Recipes

Unless noted otherwise, the recipes below serve one. Because I'm a big fan of cooking once and eating twice (or thrice), many of the recipes make multiple servings that can either be family sized or frozen for future use. If you batch cook a few of these recipes once or twice per week, you'll have a decent inventory of leftovers either in your fridge or freezer. And herein lies the secret to your success as a modern cavewoman: ready-to-go meals that meet all Paleo criteria. Bon appétit!

BREAKFAST AND SMOOTHIES

Vegetable Omelet

Sun-Dried Tomato-Pesto Omelet

Basil Pesto

Eggs and Chorizo Scramble

Scrambled Eggs Topped with Avocado and Salsa

Smoked Salmon Egg Scramble

Paleo Blueberry Pancakes

Spinach Frittata

Steak and Eggs with Tomatoes

Eggs Benedict with Orange Slices

Hollandaise Sauce

Crustless Mini-Quiche

Banana-Walnut Pancakes with Turkey Sausage

Big Breakfast

Almond Butter Dreams Smoothie

Banana Boom Protein Smoothie

Berry Blast Smoothie

Brownie Surprise

Chocolate-Strawberry Smoothie

Creamsicle Smoothie

PB & J Smoothie

Piña Colada Smoothie

Pumpkin Pie Smoothie

Tropical Smoothie

You're Makin' Me Bananas Smoothie

VEGETABLE OMELET

Serves 2

1 tablespoon extra-virgin olive oil

2 cups spinach leaves, torn

2 mushrooms, sliced

¼ bell pepper, stemmed, seeded, and diced

¼ onion, diced

3 large eggs plus 3 egg whites, beaten

In large skillet, heat olive oil over low-medium heat. Add spinach, mushrooms, pepper, and onions, and cook until tender. Remove vegetables to plate. Add eggs to skillet, stirring until lightly cooked. Add vegetables, fold omelet in half, and cook until firm.

SUN-DRIED TOMATO-PESTO OMELET

Serves 2

1 tablespoon extra-virgin olive oil

3 large eggs, beaten

¼ cup sun-dried tomatoes, chopped

2 tablespoons pesto

In skillet, heat olive oil over medium heat. Add eggs to skillet and cook until desired doneness. Add tomatoes and pesto and fold in half before serving.

BASIL PESTO

2 cups packed fresh basil leaves

3 garlic cloves, minced

⅓ cup pine nuts, cashews, or walnuts

½ cup extra-virgin olive oil

Salt and pepper to taste

Put the basil, garlic, and nuts in food processor and pulse until everything is chopped. Add the olive oil and pulse again until smooth. Season to taste with salt and pepper. Use immediately or freeze leftovers in ice cube trays and thaw individual cubes as needed.

EGGS AND CHORIZO SCRAMBLE

Serves 2

1 tablespoon coconut oil

½ onion, diced

½ red pepper, diced

½ green pepper, diced

½ pound organic chorizo, thinly sliced

4 large eggs, beaten

Hot pepper sauce, optional

Heat coconut oil in skillet. Add onions and peppers and sauté for 2 to 3 minutes. Add chorizo and cook until crispy around edges. Add eggs and scramble to mix with other ingredients until cooked to desired doneness. Serve with hot sauce, if desired.

SCRAMBLED EGGS TOPPED WITH AVOCADO AND SALSA

Serves 2

1 tablespoon coconut oil

3 large eggs, scrambled

½ avocado, scooped from skin, pit removed

1 tablespoon salsa

Place coconut oil in 9-inch skillet over medium heat until pan is evenly heated. Add in eggs and scramble. Plate and top with ½ an avocado and 1 tablespoon salsa.

SMOKED SALMON EGG SCRAMBLE

Serves 2

1 tablespoon extra-virgin olive oil

4 large eggs

4 ounces smoked salmon, diced

¼ cup chives or parsley, chopped

In skillet, heat oil over medium heat. Beat the eggs and salmon in bowl. Add the egg-salmon mixture to skillet and cook until light and fluffy. Remove from heat and sprinkle with chives before serving.

PALEO BLUEBERRY PANCAKES

Makes twelve 3-inch pancakes

1 cup almond flour
½ cup unsweetened
  applesauce
2 large eggs
¼ cup water
¼ teaspoon ground
  cinnamon

¼ teaspoon sea salt
1 cup fresh or frozen
  blueberries
1 to 2 tablespoons coconut
  oil

Combine all ingredients in bowl except blueberries and oil. Mix until thoroughly blended together. Gently fold blueberries into mixture. Heat 1 tablespoon coconut oil in large skillet over medium heat. Drop batter into pan by tablespoonful. Turn when small bubbles appear on surface of pancake. Cook evenly on both sides. Add more coconut oil to skillet to cook additional pancakes.

SPINACH FRITTATA

Serves 2

1 tablespoon extra-virgin
  olive oil
2 cups spinach leaves
2 tablespoons sun-dried
  tomatoes, chopped

1 garlic clove, minced
6 large eggs
1 cup almond milk
Sea salt and ground black
  pepper to taste

Preheat oven to broil. Add olive oil to large skillet and warm over medium heat. Add spinach and sun-dried tomatoes until spinach is wilted. Add garlic and cook for one minute. Meanwhile, combine eggs, milk, salt, and pepper in small bowl. Add mixture to pan and cook until eggs are firm. Put skillet under preheated broiler and cook until top is brown, about 3 to 5 minutes.

STEAK AND EGGS WITH TOMATOES

4 ounces hanger steak, sliced into ½-inch pieces
¼ teaspoon sea salt
¼ teaspoon ground black pepper

2 teaspoons coconut oil
¼ cup onions, diced
2 large eggs
1 large beefsteak tomato, sliced

Season sliced steak with sea salt and pepper. Heat 1 teaspoon of coconut oil in skillet and sauté onions until translucent. Add steak and cook until desired tenderness; 4 minutes per side will yield a medium-rare steak. Remove from heat and set aside on plate. In separate skillet, heat 1 teaspoon coconut oil and fry the eggs.

Remove from heat and serve with steak and tomato slices.

EGGS BENEDICT WITH ORANGE SLICES

Serves 2

Eggs Benedict

4 slices Canadian bacon
4 large eggs

2 oranges, sliced

In skillet, cook bacon until thoroughly heated. Remove from heat and set aside. Do not discard bacon fat. Add eggs and cook sunny-side up. Divide bacon among 4 plates. Place 1 egg over each slice of bacon. Top with 2 tablespoons hollandaise sauce. Garnish with orange slices.

Hollandaise Sauce

2 large egg yolks
2 tablespoons water
⅓ cup Kerrygold butter or ghee, melted
1 tablespoon fresh lemon juice

¼ teaspoon Dijon mustard
¼ teaspoon sea salt
½ teaspoon ground black pepper

Whisk egg yolks and water in small metal bowl until smooth and frothy. Place bowl over double boiler on low heat, continuously whisking eggs until they thicken. Remove from heat and continue to whisk. Whisk in butter, lemon juice, mustard, salt, and pepper; mix together well. Serve warm over eggs.

CRUSTLESS MINI-QUICHE

Serves 2

4 large eggs
2 slices cooked bacon or ham, crumbled
1 green bell pepper, seeded and diced

1 red bell pepper, seeded and diced
1 teaspoon melted coconut oil, for oiling ramekins
¼ cantaloupe, cut in half

In medium bowl, whisk eggs. Add ham or bacon and peppers and mix well. Divide egg mixture between 4 greased ramekins. Bake at 350°F for 20 minutes or until eggs are firm to touch. Gently run a knife around the edges of ramekin to remove eggs. Serve with cantaloupe wedges. (Each serving is 2 ramekins.)

BANANA-WALNUT PANCAKES WITH TURKEY SAUSAGE

Serves 4
(makes twelve 3-inch pancakes; 1 serving is 3 pancakes and 2 sausages)

1 ripe banana	¼ cup water
1 cup almond flour	¼ cup walnuts, chopped
½ cup unsweetened applesauce	2 tablespoons coconut oil plus 1 teaspoon
2 large eggs	8 turkey sausages

Combine all ingredients except coconut oil in bowl and mix until well blended. In large skillet, heat 2 tablespoons coconut oil over medium heat. Drop batter into skillet, using ¼ cup batter per pancake, and cook until small bubbles begin to form on surface. Flip pancakes and cook until done. While pancakes are cooking, split open two sausages and cook in one teaspoon coconut oil, about 2 minutes per side.

BIG BREAKFAST

1 tablespoon coconut oil	½ cup tomatoes, chopped
4 ounces ground bison	Sea salt and ground black pepper to taste
1 cup broccoli, chopped	
½ cup red onion, chopped	

In medium skillet, heat coconut oil over medium heat. Add bison, broccoli, onions, and tomatoes, and cook until meat is browned and vegetables are soft. Add salt and pepper to taste; serve immediately.

Smoothies

Smoothies are perfect for breakfast or a morning and/or afternoon snack. All smoothie recipes make one serving.

ALMOND BUTTER DREAMS SMOOTHIE

8 ounces almond milk
1 tablespoon almond
   butter

1 scoop chocolate whey
   protein powder
1 cup ice

Place all ingredients in blender and blend well.

BANANA BOOM PROTEIN SMOOTHIE

8 ounces almond milk
½ frozen banana

1 scoop vanilla protein
   powder

Place all ingredients in blender and blend well.

BERRY BLAST SMOOTHIE

8 ounces almond milk
1 cup frozen berries
   (strawberries,
   blueberries,
   raspberries)

1 scoop vanilla whey
   protein powder

Place all ingredients in blender and blend well.

BROWNIE SURPRISE

1 cup coconut milk

1 scoop chocolate whey
protein powder

1 tablespoon unsweetened
cocoa powder

¼ cup walnuts

1 cup ice

Place all ingredients in blender and blend well.

CHOCOLATE-STRAWBERRY SMOOTHIE

8 ounces unsweetened
almond milk

1 cup frozen strawberries

2 scoops chocolate whey
protein powder

Place all ingredients in blender and blend well.

CREAMSICLE SMOOTHIE

4 ounces water

4 ounces orange juice

1 scoop vanilla whey
protein powder

½ frozen banana

1 cup ice

Place all ingredients in blender and blend well.

PB & J SMOOTHIE

8 ounces almond milk
1 tablespoon almond
   butter

½ cup frozen strawberries
1 scoop vanilla whey
   protein powder

Place all ingredients in blender and blend well.

PIÑA COLADA SMOOTHIE

1 cup (unsweetened)
   coconut milk
¼ cup frozen pineapple
   chunks

2 teaspoons shredded
   coconut
1 scoop vanilla whey
   protein powder

Place all ingredients in blender and blend well.

PUMPKIN PIE SMOOTHIE

8 ounces almond milk
2 tablespoons canned
   pumpkin puree
   (unsweetened)
1 scoop vanilla whey
   protein powder

½ teaspoon ground
   cinnamon
¼ teaspoon ground
   nutmeg
1 cup ice

Place all ingredients in blender and blend well.

TROPICAL SMOOTHIE

1 cup coconut milk
½ frozen banana

1 scoop whey protein
   powder
1 teaspoon coconut flakes

Place all ingredients in blender and mix well.

YOU'RE MAKIN' ME BANANAS SMOOTHIE

8 ounces almond milk
1 frozen banana
1 scoop chocolate whey
   protein powder

1 tablespoon unsweetened
   cocoa powder

Place all ingredients in blender and mix well.

Lunch

Roasted Chicken Breasts with Arugula and Fennel Salad

Paleo Chicken Fingers and Zucchini Sticks

Apple-Walnut Chicken Salad

Paleo Mayonnaise

Grilled Chicken, Spinach, and Strawberry Salad

Chef's Salad

Curried Chicken Salad

Southwestern Turkey Burgers

Green Salad

Taco Salad

Grilled Skirt Steak with Spinach, Cranberries, and Walnuts Salad

Grilled Skirt Steak and Beet Salad

Skirt Steak with Guasaca Sauce

Grilled Steak Salad with Tangerines and Almonds

Burgers and Sweet Potato Fries

Twice-Baked Sweet Potato Skins with Bison, Spinach, and Turkey Bacon

Cajun Baked Pork Chops

Lamb Chops and Broccoli Rabe

Lamb and Greek Salad

Grilled Wild Alaskan Salmon and Spinach Salad

Chili-Seared Sea Scallops with Sautéed Watercress

Citrus Tilapia Salad

Buffalo Chicken Salad

Salmon Burgers

Crab Cakes with Paleo Aïoli

ROASTED CHICKEN BREASTS WITH ARUGULA AND FENNEL SALAD

Serves 4

1 medium fennel, thinly sliced

1 large red onion, thinly sliced

1 pound boneless, skinless chicken breasts

1 teaspoon sea salt

¼ teaspoon crushed red pepper flakes

1 cup chicken broth

2 teaspoons extra-virgin olive oil

2 cups arugula

Preheat oven to 425°F. Place fennel and onion in bottom of roasting pan and place chicken on top. Rub salt and pepper on chicken. Add chicken broth and roast until chicken is cooked, about 20 minutes. Reduce heat to 400°F and roast fennel and onions until caramelized, about 35 to 40 minutes more. Remove chicken and vegetables from roasting pan and set aside. Set roasting pan on stovetop; add olive oil and arugula. Cook 1–3 minutes over medium heat, until arugula just begins to wilt. Remove from pan and plate arugula. Top with fennel and chicken breasts.

PALEO CHICKEN FINGERS AND ZUCCHINI STICKS

Serves 4

Chicken Fingers

2 large eggs
1 cup almond flour
1 teaspoon garlic
    salt

1 teaspoon ground black
    pepper
1 pound organic chicken
    strips

Preheat oven to 350°F. Beat large eggs in shallow bowl. Mix almond flour, garlic salt, and pepper in another shallow bowl. Dredge chicken strips on both sides in egg mixture, and then almond flour mixture to coat. Arrange chicken strips on baking sheet and bake 20 minutes or until edges are crispy.

Zucchini Sticks

4 medium zucchini, cut
    into thin strips (the size
    of French fries)

1 tablespoon extra-virgin
    olive oil
1 teaspoon sea salt

Preheat oven to 350°F. Place zucchini sticks on parchment paper–lined baking sheet. Toss with olive oil and sea salt. Bake until lightly browned, turning once with a spatula, about 25 minutes.

APPLE-WALNUT CHICKEN SALAD

4 ounces grilled chicken, chopped

2 cups spinach

½ cup walnuts

½ cup apple, chopped

1 tablespoon Paleo Mayonnaise (see recipe below)

2 tablespoons balsamic vinegar

Place all items in bowl, toss, and serve.

Paleo Mayonnaise

1 large egg

1 teaspoon lemon juice

¼ teaspoon mustard powder

½ cup extra-virgin olive oil

1 teaspoon apple cider vinegar

Place egg, lemon juice, and mustard powder in bowl and whisk until well blended. Add in olive oil and vinegar, and keep whisking until it forms consistency of mayonnaise. Store in refrigerator; will keep up to 5 days.

GRILLED CHICKEN, SPINACH, AND STRAWBERRY SALAD

4 ounces chicken breast, grilled and sliced
1 cup spinach leaves
4 strawberries, sliced
1 tablespoon almonds, slivered
2 tablespoons balsamic vinegar
1 tablespoon extra-virgin olive oil

Mix salad ingredients together in small bowl. Drizzle with vinegar and olive oil. Toss and serve.

CHEF'S SALAD

Serves 4

1 head romaine lettuce
4 large eggs, hard boiled and sliced
1 cup grilled chicken, diced
1 cup cooked turkey, diced
1 cucumber, diced
2 slices bacon, diced
1 tablespoon extra-virgin olive oil
2 tablespoons balsamic vinegar

Place all ingredients in bowl, toss, and serve.

CURRIED CHICKEN SALAD

Serves 2

2 cups cooked chicken
breasts, chopped
¼ cup raisins
1 carrot, shredded
½ cup celery, chopped
1 tablespoon Paleo
Mayonnaise
1 tablespoon lemon juice

1 teaspoon curry powder
1 tablespoon fresh parsley,
chopped
¼ teaspoon sea salt
½ teaspoon ground black
pepper
2 cups baby lettuce greens

Combine all ingredients in bowl except greens and mix well. Serve chicken salad on greens.

SOUTHWESTERN TURKEY BURGERS

Serves 3 to 4

1 pound organic turkey
meat
½ cup tomatoes, diced
¼ cup cilantro, chopped
¼ cup scallions, finely
chopped

¼ cup red or yellow
bell peppers, finely
chopped
¼ teaspoon sea salt

Combine all ingredients in bowl and mix thoroughly. Divide into 4 equal portions and shape each portion into ½-inch-thick burgers. Grill burgers for 3 to 4 minutes per side or until desired doneness at 400°F.

GREEN SALAD

Serves 4

1 garlic clove, halved
1 teaspoon Dijon
  mustard
1 tablespoon balsamic
  vinegar

Sea salt and ground black
  pepper to taste
3 tablespoons extra-virgin
  olive oil
4 cups mixed greens

Rub inside of large bowl with garlic halves and then run them through garlic press. Add crushed garlic, mustard, and vinegar to bowl and whisk vigorously for about 10 seconds. Season with salt and pepper to taste. Drizzle in olive oil as slowly as possible with one hand while whisking as quickly as possible with the other hand to emulsify. Toss salad greens with dressing just before serving.

TACO SALAD

Serves 4

1 tablespoon grapeseed oil
1 pound ground organic
  bison or turkey
1 packet Simply Organic
  Spicy Taco Seasoning
2 cups romaine lettuce,
  chopped

2 medium tomatoes,
  chopped
½ sweet onion, chopped
1 medium cucumber,
  seeded, peeled, and
  chopped
1 cup black olives, sliced

Heat grapeseed oil in large skillet over medium heat. Add bison and cook, breaking up with a wooden spoon until lightly browned. Add seasoning packet and mix well. Cook, stirring, until bison is fully cooked. Remove from heat. Divide lettuce, tomatoes, onions, cucumbers, and olives among four bowls. Top with taco meat and serve with a dollop of guacamole if desired.

GRILLED SKIRT STEAK WITH SPINACH, CRANBERRIES, AND WALNUTS SALAD

Serves 2

1 pound skirt steak	Spinach
1 tablespoon extra-virgin olive oil	2 tablespoons cranberries, chopped
2 garlic cloves, run through a garlic press	2 tablespoons walnuts, chopped
1 teaspoon sea salt	1 tablespoon balsamic vinegar
1 teaspoon ground black pepper	

Preheat grill or grill pan. Rub steaks with olive oil. Distribute garlic evenly between 2 steaks and rub on both sides well. Season with salt and pepper. Grill steaks for 4 minutes per side at 375°F for medium-rare or until desired doneness. Serve atop handful of spinach leaves sprinkled with cranberries, walnuts, and vinegar.

GRILLED SKIRT STEAK AND BEET SALAD

Serves 2

1 pound beets, tops
    removed and 1-inch
    stems left attached
1 pound skirt steak
1 tablespoon extra-virgin
    olive oil

⅓ cup cilantro, chopped
2 tablespoons red wine
    vinegar
½ teaspoon sea salt

Preheat oven to 475°F. Wrap beets individually in aluminum foil and place on baking sheet. Roast beets until they can be pierced with a knife, about 45 to 60 minutes. Remove from oven and let cool. Peel off skins and cut into ½-inch chunks.

Rub beef with olive oil. Place steak in ovenproof baking dish and roast for 12 minutes. Let sit for 5 minutes and cut into 1-inch cubes. Place all ingredients in bowl; add cilantro, vinegar, and salt. Serve immediately.

SKIRT STEAK WITH GUASACA SAUCE

Serves 2

1 small, ripe avocado
½ cup cilantro
2 tablespoons onion,
    chopped
1 small garlic clove,
    minced
1 tablespoon rice vinegar
1 to 2 tablespoons fresh
    lime juice

1 to 2 teaspoons jalapeño
1 cup water
½ cup coconut milk
Sea salt to taste
12 ounces skirt steak
1 teaspoon extra-virgin
    olive oil
1 teaspoon ground black
    pepper

Preheat broiler. Put avocado, cilantro, onion, garlic, vinegar, lime juice, and jalapeño in food processor and process until smooth. Slowly add water and milk until sauce is thin. Taste sauce for seasoning, adding more as necessary.

Rub steak with olive oil, pepper, and salt. Broil 4 minutes per side for medium-rare. Cut steak in half and serve.

GRILLED STEAK SALAD WITH TANGERINES AND ALMONDS

4 ounces flank steak
1 tablespoon chili powder
1 teaspoon extra-virgin olive oil
2 limes, juiced
½ bag mixed green salad
¼ cup orange juice
1 teaspoon extra-virgin olive oil

2 tablespoons balsamic vinegar
Sea salt and ground black pepper to taste
2 tangerines, peeled and segmented
¼ cup almonds, sliced

Rub chili powder, 1 teaspoon olive oil, and juice of limes on both sides of steak. Cook steak in grill pan over medium-high heat; 4 minutes per side will yield a medium-rare piece. Cut into slices. Place mixed greens in bowl and put steak slices on top. In separate small bowl mix orange juice, olive oil, balsamic vinegar, salt, and pepper. Pour mixture over steak salad. Top with tangerines segments and almond slices. Toss and serve.

BURGERS AND SWEET POTATO FRIES

Serves 4

Sweet Potato Fries

2 sweet potatoes, peeled   1 tablespoon extra-virgin
   and cut lengthwise into   olive oil
   ¼ pieces   1 teaspoon sea salt

Preheat oven to 325°F. Peel and slice 2 sweet potatoes into ¼-inch strips. In large bowl, toss sweet potatoes with olive oil and sea salt to coat thoroughly. Arrange potatoes in single layer on foil-lined baking sheet. Bake until sweet potatoes are lightly browned and crispy, turning once halfway, about 30 minutes.

Burgers

1 pound lean ground beef,   ¼ teaspoon paprika
   turkey, or bison   ½ teaspoon garlic powder
½ teaspoon sea salt   1 teaspoon dried parsley

In medium bowl, combine meat, sea salt, paprika, and garlic powder with your (clean) hands. Divide into 4 portions. Flatten into patties about ½-inch thick. Heat stove-top grill pan over medium heat; cook burgers 3 minutes per side.

TWICE-BAKED SWEET POTATO SKINS WITH BISON, SPINACH, AND TURKEY BACON

Serves 2

2 sweet potatoes
1 tablespoon extra-virgin
   olive oil
½ onion, diced
8 ounces ground bison

1 cup spinach leaves,
   chopped
2 pieces cooked turkey
   bacon, chopped
2 garlic cloves, minced

Bake pierced sweet potatoes at 350°F for 1 hour. Remove from oven but keep oven on. When cool enough to handle, cut in half and scoop out flesh. Reserve skins.

While potatoes are cooking, heat the olive oil in a large skillet. Add the onions and sauté until translucent, about 5 minutes. Add garlic and ground bison and cook until browned. Add spinach and cook until wilted. Add bison mixture to sweet potato flesh and mix together. Spoon bison mixture back into scooped-out potato skins. Sprinkle with chopped turkey bacon pieces. Return to oven and bake for 10 to 15 minutes, until potato skins are crisp.

CAJUN BAKED PORK CHOPS

Serves 2

Two 6-ounce center-cut
   loin pork chops

1 tablespoon Cajun
   seasoning

Preheat oven to 350°F. Rub Cajun seasoning into pork chops. Arrange pork chops in baking dish and bake for 30 minutes or until instant-read thermometer inserted into center reads 150°F.

LAMB CHOPS AND BROCCOLI RABE

Serves 2

Two 6-ounce veal chops
1 tablespoon Dijon
    mustard

1 bunch broccoli rabe
1 tablespoon unsalted
    butter

Preheat oven to broil. Place lamb chops on broiling pan; brush both sides with mustard. Broil 6 to 8 minutes per side, depending on desired doneness.

Trim bottoms from 1 bunch broccoli rabe. In skillet, heat 1 tablespoon butter over medium heat until melted. Add broccoli rabe and cover. Cook about 3 minutes or until color is bright green and texture is al dente.

LAMB AND GREEK SALAD

Serves 2

½ cup organic beef broth
1 tablespoon Dijon mustard
2 tablespoons fresh lemon
    juice
1 garlic clove, minced
8 ounces boneless lamb
    sirloin or chops, cut
    into cubes
1 tablespoon extra-virgin
    olive oil
1 tablespoon water
⅛ teaspoon sea salt

⅛ teaspoon ground black
    pepper
1 tablespoon scallions,
    sliced
1 small tomato, diced
½ cucumber, diced
5 Kalamata olives,
    chopped
1 cup romaine lettuce,
    chopped

Mix broth, mustard, 1 tablespoon lemon juice, and garlic in shallow dish. Add lamb to marinade. Cover and refrigerate for 4 hours, turning once. Preheat grill or broiler. Grill or broil on high heat for 4 minutes per side.

In small bowl, whisk oil, water, remaining 1 tablespoon lemon juice, salt, and pepper. Add scallions, tomatoes, cucumbers, and olives, and toss to coat well. Pour mixture on top of romaine lettuce and toss. Top with grilled lamb chops.

GRILLED WILD ALASKAN SALMON AND SPINACH SALAD

Serves 2 generously

1 pound skinless wild salmon fillet	⅛ teaspoon ground black pepper
2 teaspoons extra-virgin olive oil	2 cups fresh spinach leaves
⅛ teaspoon sea salt	1 lemon, halved

Heat large skillet over medium heat. Rub salmon on both sides with olive oil; sprinkle with salt and pepper. Place salmon in skillet pan over medium-high heat and cook until center is opaque, about 4 minutes on each side. Divide spinach in 2 serving bowls, squeeze half of the lemon on each bowl of spinach, and toss. Place cooked salmon and pan juices on top of each bowl of spinach.

CHILI-SEARED SEA SCALLOPS WITH SAUTÉED WATERCRESS

Serves 2

3 tablespoons fresh lemon juice

2 teaspoons chili powder

½ teaspoon lemon zest

½ teaspoon ground cumin

½ teaspoon sea salt

¼ teaspoon cayenne pepper

¾ pound sea scallops

2 tablespoons extra-virgin olive oil

4 garlic cloves, minced

2 bunches watercress

1 teaspoon sea salt

¼ cup chicken broth

Whisk together lemon juice, chili powder, lemon zest, cumin, salt, and cayenne in small bowl. Add scallops to mixture and toss to coat; let sit for 15 minutes. In large skillet, add 1 tablespoon olive oil and place heat on low to medium. Place scallops in skillet, turning scallops until they are golden brown on outside and just opaque in center, about 2 minutes on each side. Remove from skillet and set aside.

In same skillet, heat 1 tablespoon olive oil. Add garlic and sauté for 30 seconds. Add watercress and salt. Cook, tossing continuously, until wilted. Add chicken broth, cover, and simmer for 1 minute. Serve immediately.

CITRUS TILAPIA SALAD

Serves 2

Two 6-ounce tilapia filets
½ teaspoon sea salt
½ teaspoon ground black
  pepper
½ cup fresh orange juice
2 teaspoons garlic powder
2 tablespoons extra-virgin
  olive oil

1 cup celery, chopped
1 cup carrots, chopped
2 cup mixed salad greens
2 clementine oranges,
  peeled and segmented
½ cup almonds

Preheat broiler. Season both sides of tilapia with 1 teaspoon olive oil, salt, and pepper. Put fish in shallow roasting pan. Drizzle with 1 tablespoon orange juice; sprinkle with garlic powder. Broil fish for 4 to 5 minutes. In large bowl, combine celery, carrots, greens, clementines, and almonds. Add remaining olive oil and orange juice; toss well. Arrange salad on 2 plates and top with fish.

BUFFALO CHICKEN SALAD

Serves 4

1 pound chicken tenders
½ cup hot sauce (with
  no added sugar or
  preservatives)
2 bunches spinach
1 large cucumber, chopped
1 pint cherry tomatoes,
  halved

2 carrots, chopped
1 tablespoon olive oil
1 tablespoon balsamic
  vinegar

Preheat oven to 350°F. Line baking sheet with parchment paper and set aside. Brush chicken tenders with hot pepper sauce on both sides. Place chicken on lined baking sheet and bake 25 minutes. Place chicken atop salad of spinach, cucumbers, tomatoes, and carrots. Drizzle with olive oil and balsamic vinegar.

SALMON BURGERS

Serves 2

One 12-ounce can wild Alaskan salmon, drained
2 teaspoons Dijon mustard
1 large egg
½ onion, chopped
1 tablespoon almond flour
Juice of ½ lemon
2 tablespoons parsley, chopped
1 tablespoon coconut oil

Mix salmon, Dijon mustard, egg, onions, almond flour, lemon, and parsley together in bowl. Shape mixture into 4 small burgers.

Heat coconut oil in large skillet over medium heat. Add burgers and sauté in pan for 4 minutes each side, or bake in oven for 15 minutes at 350°F.

CRAB CAKES WITH PALEO AÏOLI

Serves 2

Crab Cakes

6 ounces lump crabmeat, picked over and chopped
¼ cup celery, finely diced
¼ cup onion, finely diced
1 large egg, beaten
2 tablespoons Dijon mustard

½ teaspoon Old Bay
  seasoning
2 tablespoons coconut
  milk
2 tablespoons coconut
  flour

1 tablespoon parsley,
  chopped
½ teaspoon sea salt
½ teaspoon ground black
  pepper
2 tablespoons coconut oil

Combine all ingredients except coconut oil in bowl. Shape mixture into small patties. Heat coconut oil in medium skillet and sauté crab cakes for about 4 minutes on each side. Serve with a dollop of aïoli on the side.

Paleo Aïoli

2 egg yolks
2 teaspoons fresh lemon
  juice
2 garlic cloves, minced

¼ teaspoon dry mustard
½ cup extra-virgin olive oil
1 teaspoon white vinegar

Place egg yolks, lemon juice, garlic, and mustard in bowl and whisk until well blended. Add olive oil and vinegar and keep whisking until it forms consistency of mayonnaise. Store in airtight container or jar in refrigerator; will keep up to 5 days.

DINNER

Roasted Chicken and Green Beans

Pesto Chicken and Roasted Broccoli

"Bruschetta" Chicken, Roasted Acorn Squash, and Sautéed Asparagus

Chicken Rolled with Broccoli Rabe and Sun-Dried Tomatoes

Pecan-Crusted Chicken with Sautéed Asparagus and Butternut Squash Soup

Stir-Fried Chicken and Vegetables

Spaghetti Squash with Italian Chicken Sausage and Steamed Broccoli

Turkey Chili and Steamed Spinach

Turkey Meatballs with Spaghetti Squash and Steamed Broccoli

Lettuce Wrap Turkey Tacos and Butternut Squash Soup

Turkey-Vegetable Lasagna

Mama's Sunday Meatballs and Spaghetti Squash

Skirt Steak with Roasted Asparagus, Sweet Potato, and Onion

Skirt Steak with Chimichurri Sauce, Cherry Tomatoes, and Sweet Potato Skewers

Pepper Steak with Peppers and Onions

Filet Mignon and Broccoli Rabe

Zucchini Pasta with Meat Sauce

Stuffed Peppers

Grilled Wild Salmon with Pesto

Sweet Potato–Crusted Wild Salmon

Cajun Catfish, Mashed Parsnips and Apples, and Roasted Brussels Sprouts

Almond-Crusted Tilapia and Sweet Potato Mash

Fish Tacos

Sesame Seared Tuna with Seaweed Salad

Coconut Shrimp with Sesame Bok Choy

Grilled Rosemary-Garlic Shrimp with Grilled Vegetables

Cucumber Sushi and Wasabi Mashed "Potatoes"

ROASTED CHICKEN AND GREEN BEANS

Serves 4 to 6

Roasted Chicken

One 4- to 5-pound chicken

2 tablespoons butter, clarified

1 tablespoon garlic powder

1 tablespoon onion powder

1 tablespoon powdered sage

Sea salt to taste

Ground black pepper to taste

2 sprigs thyme

Preheat oven to 375°F. Rinse chicken and pat dry with paper towels; place breast side up in roasting pan. Rub chicken inside and out with melted butter, and then sprinkle on garlic powder, onion powder, sage powder, salt, and pepper. Put thyme sprigs in cavity. Roast for 75 minutes or until instant-read thermometer registers 160°F at thickest part of thigh. Remove from oven and let chicken rest for 10 to 15 minutes before carving.

Green Beans

½ pound green beans
1 tablespoon butter, clarified

Fill 2-quart saucepan ¾ full with water. Bring to boil. Add green beans and cook for 3 minutes, until bright green in color. Drain green beans in colander and place in bowl of ice water for 30 seconds to stop further cooking and retain green color. Just before serving, reheat green beans and add butter to pot; toss well before serving.

PESTO CHICKEN AND ROASTED BROCCOLI

Serves 2

Two 6-ounce chicken breasts
1 teaspoon olive oil
Basil Pesto (see recipe, page 198)

Arrange chicken breasts in baking dish and rub with extra-virgin olive oil. Bake at 350°F for 25 minutes.

Arrange cooked chicken on plates and top each breast with 1 tablespoon pesto; serve with roasted broccoli.

Roasted Broccoli

2 bunches organic
broccoli, cut into large
florets
5 tablespoons olive oil
1 ½ teaspoons sea salt

½ teaspoon freshly ground
pepper
4 garlic cloves, peeled and
diced
1 whole lemon

Preheat oven to 425°F. Wash and thoroughly dry broccoli florets; otherwise they will be more soggy than crispy when baked. Place the broccoli on a cookie sheet. Toss with olive oil, sea salt, pepper and garlic. Roast in the oven 20 to 25 minutes, until crisp-tender and lightly browned. Remove from heat and set aside. Zest the lemon over the broccoli and then cut in half, remove seeds, and squeeze the lemon juice over the broccoli. Serve immediately.

"BRUSCHETTA" CHICKEN, ROASTED ACORN SQUASH, AND SAUTÉED ASPARAGUS

Serves 4

"Bruschetta" Chicken

1 pound boneless, skinless
chicken cutlets
1 tablespoon plus one
teaspoon extra-virgin
olive oil
4 tomatoes, diced

¼ cup red onion, diced
12 basil leaves
1 garlic clove, minced
Sea salt and ground black
pepper to taste

Preheat oven to 350°F. Rub chicken with 1 tablespoon of the olive oil; place in 9 x 13–inch baking dish. Bake chicken for 15 to 20 minutes, or until center is opaque and juices run clear. Mix all the ingredients for bruschetta and the remaining teaspoon of olive oil together in bowl. Spoon bruschetta mixture over cooked chicken and serve.

Roasted Acorn Squash

2 medium acorn squash, cut in half and seeded
1 teaspoon extra-virgin olive oil

2 teaspoons ground cinnamon

Preheat oven to 400°F. Place acorn squash halves, cut side up, in baking dish. Brush olive oil and cinnamon on top of squash. Roast squash until tender, about 30 minutes, and serve.

Sautéed Asparagus

1 bunch asparagus
1 teaspoon extra-virgin olive oil

1 teaspoon butter

Take asparagus and wash well; pat dry. Trim off ½ inch from base of asparagus stalks.

Heat olive oil and butter in large skillet over medium heat. Once butter is melted, add asparagus and cover. Give a toss after 2 minutes, and cook another 2 to 3 minutes or until asparagus is al dente and a vibrant green color.

CHICKEN ROLLED WITH BROCCOLI
RABE AND SUN-DRIED TOMATOES

Serves 4

1 tablespoon extra-virgin olive oil

4 garlic cloves, chopped

½ cup onions, diced

1 bunch broccoli rabe, ends trimmed

1 pound chicken cutlets, pounded flat

1 cup sun-dried tomatoes

1 cup organic free-range chicken stock

1 cup fresh tomatoes, diced

In large saucepan, heat olive oil. Add garlic, onions, and broccoli rabe, and cook until broccoli rabe is bright green and al dente. Remove from heat and set aside.

Preheat oven to 350°F. Lay chicken cutlets on flat surface. Place 2 to 3 stalks broccoli rabe, onions, and garlic on top of each chicken breast and top with sun-dried tomatoes. Roll up each chicken breast and place seam side down in baking dish. Add chicken broth. Place diced tomatoes and remaining juices from cooked broccoli rabe on top of chicken. Bake for 30 minutes.

PECAN-CRUSTED CHICKEN WITH SAUTÉED ASPARAGUS AND BUTTERNUT SQUASH SOUP

Chicken and asparagus serves 4; soup serves 6

Butternut Squash Soup

3 pounds butternut squash, halved and seeds scooped out

6 cups organic reduced-sodium chicken broth

1 medium parsnip, peeled and cut into ½-inch slices

1 medium Granny Smith apple, peeled, cored, and chopped

¼ cup coconut milk, unsweetened

½ teaspoon sea salt

2 tablespoons chives, chopped

Preheat oven to 350°F. Place squash halves cut side down in baking dish. Bake 45 minutes to 1 hour or until flesh gives easily when pierced with knife. Remove from heat and set aside. When cool enough to handle, use spoon and scoop out flesh. Place squash in blender with 4 cups chicken broth. Blend until pureed. Pour soup into pot and add remaining 2 cups chicken broth, parsnips, and apples; bring to boil. Reduce heat and simmer; cook until parsnips and apples are soft. Stir in coconut milk and salt, and remove from heat. Garnish with chives and serve hot. This soup is even better the next day and freezes well in glass container for 4 months. (You will have plenty left over.)

Pecan-Crusted Chicken

1 large egg

2 teaspoons unsweetened almond milk

1 cup pecans, chopped

½ teaspoon ground black pepper

1 tablespoon parsley, chopped

Four 6-ounce chicken breasts

2 teaspoons extra-virgin olive oil

Preheat oven to 350°F. In medium bowl, beat egg and almond milk and set aside. In separate bowl, combine chopped pecans, pepper, and parsley. Dip chicken breasts into egg mixture and coat on both sides, and then press chicken breasts into pecan mixture to coat fully.

Arrange chicken in shallow baking pan coated with olive oil and bake 20 minutes or until fully cooked.

Sautéed Asparagus (see page 230 for recipe).

STIR-FRIED CHICKEN AND VEGETABLES

Serves 4

1 tablespoon coconut oil

1 pound chicken tenders

½ onion, chopped

1 garlic clove, minced

1 red pepper, seeded and sliced

1 green pepper, seeded and sliced

1 cup snap peas, trimmed

One 8-ounce can sliced water chestnuts, rinsed and drained

¼ cup red wine

Heat coconut oil in skillet or wok over high heat. Add chicken, turning often, until chicken is almost cooked; remove from skillet and set aside. Add the onions and garlic to skillet and sauté until onions are translucent. Add vegetables and sauté all ingredients together. Add the chicken back to the skillet, along with the wine. Cook on low for 5 minutes until the sauce begins to reduce.

SPAGHETTI SQUASH WITH ITALIAN CHICKEN SAUSAGE AND STEAMED BROCCOLI

Serves 4

Spaghetti Squash

1 large spaghetti squash, cut in half lengthwise and seeds removed

Preheat oven to 375°F. Pour 2 cups water in baking dish large enough to hold squash in a single layer. Arrange squash cut side down in water. Bake 30 minutes or until squash can be pierced with a fork. Remove squash from baking dish and set aside. When cool enough to handle, scrape inside of squash with a fork; squash will come out like spaghetti. Place squash on serving platter and top with sauce before serving.

Italian Chicken Sausage

1 tablespoon extra-virgin
olive oil
4 garlic cloves, minced
1 small onion, chopped

1 pound herb-flavored
chicken sausage, sliced
into ¼-inch pieces
1 cup crushed tomatoes,
fresh or canned

Heat olive oil in skillet over medium heat; add garlic, onions, and chicken sausage and sauté until onions are translucent and garlic and sausage are lightly browned. Pour in crushed tomatoes and season with Italian seasonings. Simmer while stirring for 10 minutes and then let it sit.

Steamed Broccoli

Chop head of broccoli into bite-sized florets. Place in steamer with 1-inch water or add 1-inch water in 2-quart saucepan. Steam for 3 to 5 minutes or until bright green and fork tender.

TURKEY CHILI AND STEAMED SPINACH

Serves 4

Turkey Chili

1 teaspoon extra-virgin olive oil
½ onion, diced
1 garlic clove, minced
1 pound ground turkey
1 cup tomatoes, diced
½ teaspoon sea salt
1 teaspoon ground black pepper
1 teaspoon garlic powder
½ teaspoon chili powder

In large skillet, sauté onions and garlic in olive oil. Add turkey and stir frequently until it loses its pale color. Add tomatoes, salt, pepper, garlic powder, and chili powder. Simmer until turkey is fully cooked.

Steamed Spinach

9 ounces regular spinach, trimmed, or baby spinach
1 tablespoon extra-virgin olive oil
1 tablespoon fresh lemon juice, plus lemon wedges for garnish
⅛ teaspoon coarse salt

Fill medium saucepan with 2 inches of water, and fit with steamer insert. Bring to a boil. Add spinach. Reduce to a simmer. Cover, and steam until spinach has wilted, about 1 to 2 minutes.

Transfer to serving bowl. Toss with oil, lemon juice, and salt. Garnish with lemon. Serve immediately.

TURKEY MEATBALLS WITH SPAGHETTI
SQUASH AND STEAMED BROCCOLI

Serves 4

Turkey Meatballs

1 pound ground turkey	1 garlic clove, crushed
2 tablespoons parsley,	1 tablespoon grapeseed oil
chopped	One 32-ounce jar organic
1 teaspoon onion powder	tomato sauce

In medium bowl, combine turkey, parsley, onion powder, and garlic. Mix well and shape into 1-inch meatballs. Pour grapeseed oil in large skillet and heat over medium heat. Add meatballs and brown on both sides. Add tomato sauce and reduce heat to low; simmer for 30 minutes.

Spaghetti Squash (see recipe, page 234)

Steamed Broccoli (see recipe, page 235)

LETTUCE WRAP TURKEY TACOS AND
BUTTERNUT SQUASH SOUP

Serves 4

Lettuce Wrap Turkey Tacos

1 tablespoon coconut oil	1 packet Simply Organic
1 pound ground turkey	spicy taco seasoning

8 romaine lettuce leaves   ½ cup salsa
1 cup guacamole

In large skillet, heat coconut oil over medium heat. Brown ground turkey, stirring frequently. Add taco seasoning and mix well. Remove from heat and set aside. Break lettuce leaves apart, wash well, pat dry, and stack on plate.

Take an open lettuce leaf and top with guacamole and salsa. Roll up into wrap and serve.

Butternut Squash Soup (see recipe, page 232)

TURKEY-VEGETABLE LASAGNA

Serves 6

3 large eggplants, sliced
⅛-inch thick
3 large zucchini, sliced
⅛-inch thick
1½ teaspoons sea salt
1 tablespoon extra-virgin
olive oil
1 small onion, finely
chopped

2 garlic cloves, minced
1½ pounds ground turkey
3 large tomatoes, freshly
chopped
1 tablespoon dried basil
1 teaspoon dried oregano
¼ teaspoon ground black
pepper

Toss sliced eggplant and zucchini in large skillet with salt, tossing once or twice to coat well. Lay strips on paper towels on work surface; set aside for 1 hour. Drain off any excess water.

In large saucepan, heat olive oil and sauté onions over medium heat until translucent. Add garlic and sauté another minute. Add ground turkey and cook until browned. Stir in tomatoes, basil, oregano, and pepper. Cook, stirring occasionally, until tomatoes start to break down and sauce thickens, about 25 minutes. Remove from heat and set aside.

Preheat oven to 350°F and position rack in center of oven. Blot any moisture off zucchini and eggplant strips with paper towels. Use ⅓ eggplant to line bottom of a 9 x 13–inch baking pan, layering lengthwise like you would lasagna noodles. Place layer of zucchini strips in opposite direction and then top with ⅓ of tomato-and-turkey-meat mixture. Repeat this process two more times, ending with sauce.

Bake, uncovered, until bubbling, about 30 to 45 minutes. Let stand at room temperature for 10 minutes before serving. Slice into six pieces and serve.

MAMA'S SUNDAY MEATBALLS AND SPAGHETTI SQUASH

Serves 4

Tomato Sauce

1 tablespoon extra-virgin olive oil

3 garlic cloves, minced

1 pound canned or fresh plum tomatoes (skins removed), cut into quarters

½ teaspoon parsley, chopped

½ teaspoon dried oregano

1 teaspoon basil, chopped

¼ teaspoon sea salt

¼ teaspoon ground black pepper

In large skillet, sauté garlic in olive oil over low-medium heat until lightly browned. Add tomatoes, parsley, oregano, basil, salt, and pepper. Simmer for 20 to 30 minutes, stirring occasionally. (Prepare meatballs while sauce is cooking.)

Spaghetti Squash (see recipe, page 234)

Meatballs

1 pound ground buffalo or turkey
1 onion, grated
1 large egg
1 tablespoon parsley, chopped
1 teaspoon dried oregano
2 garlic cloves, crushed
¼ teaspoon sea salt
¼ teaspoon ground black pepper
¼ cup basil, chopped
1 tablespoon grapeseed oil

In medium bowl, use your hands to mix together all ingredients well (except grapeseed oil). Shape mixture into 1-inch balls. In skillet, heat oil over low to medium heat. Place meatballs in pan, turning as needed until brown on all sides.

Transfer meatballs to pot with tomato sauce. Simmer for additional 30 minutes. To serve, place squash on serving platter and top with meatballs and sauce.

SKIRT STEAK WITH ROASTED ASPARAGUS, SWEET POTATO, AND ONION

1 sweet potato, diced
1 onion, diced
1 tablespoon plus 1 teaspoon extra-virgin olive oil
¼ teaspoon sea salt
8 asparagus spears, trimmed
1 teaspoon sea salt
One 6-ounce skirt steak
1 teaspoon grapeseed olive oil
1 teaspoon sea salt
1 teaspoon ground black pepper

Preheat oven to 400°F. Toss sweet potatoes and onions with 1 tablespoon olive oil and sea salt in baking dish large enough to hold vegetables in single layer. Bake 45 minutes, stirring once after 25 minutes. Remove from oven and cover.

While sweet potatoes and onions are roasting, drizzle asparagus with 1 teaspoon olive oil and sea salt and place in baking dish large enough to hold vegetables in single layer. Roast 12 minutes. Serve immediately.

Heat skillet to medium-high. Rub oil, salt, and pepper into both sides of steak. Cook on high heat for about 4 minutes each side or until desired doneness.

SKIRT STEAK WITH CHIMICHURRI SAUCE, CHERRY TOMATOES, AND SWEET POTATO SKEWERS

Serves 4

Sweet Potato Skewers

2 sweet potatoes, rinsed and cut into 1-inch cubes
1 tablespoon extra-virgin olive oil
Sea salt and ground black pepper to taste

3 bamboo sticks or metal skewers (if using bamboo skewers, soak in water for 15 minutes)

Preheat oven to 400°F. Toss sweet potatoes, olive oil, salt, and pepper together to coat. Arrange sweet potatoes on skewers. Arrange skewers on baking sheet and bake for 30 minutes, or until desired doneness.

Skirt Steak

1 pound skirt steak, cut into 4 pieces	Sea salt and ground black pepper to taste
1 tablespoon extra-virgin olive oil	1 pint cherry tomatoes, sliced in half
2 garlic cloves, run through a garlic press	1 tablespoon balsamic vinegar

Preheat grill or grill pan on medium-high heat. Rinse and pat dry steak; set aside on a small platter. Generously rub steak with olive oil. Evenly distribute garlic among steaks. Season with salt and pepper. Grill for 4 minutes per side for medium-rare or until desired doneness. Toss cherry tomatoes with balsamic vinegar and serve with steak and sweet potato skewers.

Chimichurri Sauce

1 cup fresh parsley	2 tablespoons onion, chopped
1 cup fresh cilantro	½ cup extra-virgin olive oil
2 tablespoons oregano leaves	1 teaspoon fresh lime juice
½ tablespoon garlic, minced	2 tablespoons white vinegar
	1 teaspoon sea salt

Place parsley, cilantro, oregano, garlic, and onion in food processor; blend until finely chopped. Transfer to medium bowl, add olive oil, lime juice, vinegar, and sea salt; mix together. Spoon chimichurri sauce over cooked skirt steak. Sauce will keep for 1 week in refrigerator.

PEPPER STEAK WITH PEPPERS AND ONIONS

Serves 4

2 tablespoons extra-virgin
olive oil
1 pound grass-fed steak,
cut into ¼-inch slices
1 onion, thinly sliced

4 bell peppers (yellow,
orange, green, and/or
red), seeded and thinly
sliced
½ teaspoon garlic salt
½ teaspoon ground black
pepper

Heat oil in large skillet over medium-high heat. Add meat and onions and cook until onions are slightly translucent. Stir in peppers and continue to cook for another 5 minutes. Season with garlic salt and pepper.

FILET MIGNON AND BROCCOLI RABE

Serves 2

Two 8-ounce filet mignon
steaks
1 tablespoon plus 2
teaspoons extra-virgin
olive oil
3 garlic cloves, run
through a garlic press

½ teaspoon sea salt
½ teaspoon ground black
pepper
1 bunch broccoli rabe,
trimmed

Heat a large skillet over medium-high heat. Generously rub steaks with 1 tablespoon of the olive oil and garlic. Season with salt and pepper. Grill steaks for 4 minutes per side or until desired doneness. Remove from heat and set aside.

Add the remaining 2 teaspoons olive oil to same skillet. When heated, add broccoli rabe. Sauté, tossing regularly, for 5 minutes or until bright green and tender.

ZUCCHINI PASTA WITH MEAT SAUCE

Serves 6

1 tablespoon extra-virgin olive oil	One 28-ounce can tomato puree
1 carrot, finely grated	½ teaspoon sea salt
1 celery stalk, finely grated	1 bunch fresh basil
1 small onion, finely grated	2 large zucchini, peeled and ends trimmed
2 garlic cloves, minced	
1 pound ground beef and pork (½ pound each)	

Heat olive oil in large, heavy-bottomed pot over medium heat. Add carrot, celery, and onion; cover and steam, stirring every few minutes, until onions are translucent and all liquid has evaporated. Add garlic and cook another minute. Add meat and cook until browned. Add the tomato puree, salt, and basil. Cover and reduce heat to low; simmer for 30 minutes.

Place zucchini in spiralizer vegetable slicer (available at Amazon.com) set to the smallest blade. (Note: zucchini will cook and release liquid once it comes in contact with sauce. If you have time, put shredded zucchini in colander, toss with ¼ teaspoon salt, and let drain for 10 to 15 minutes. Using your hands, squeeze any excess water from zucchini.) Serve meat sauce over the zucchini.

STUFFED PEPPERS

Serves 4

4 red bell peppers, halved
and seeded

2 tablespoons extra-virgin
olive oil

1 medium onion, chopped

2 garlic cloves, minced

1 pound organic ground
bison meat

½ cup organic chicken
stock

4 cups spinach leaves,
torn

2 cups tomatoes, diced
(about 2 large)

½ teaspoon chili powder

½ teaspoon sea salt

¼ teaspoon ground black
pepper

Preheat oven to 375°F. In large pot of boiling water, cook bell peppers until tender, about 4 minutes, then drain.

For filling, heat large skillet with olive oil over medium heat. Add onion, garlic, and bison, and cook until meat is browned. Add chicken stock, spinach, tomatoes, chili powder, salt, and pepper; bring to simmer. Reduce heat and stir occasionally until all flavors are blended, about 10 minutes.

Divide filling among bell pepper halves. Place stuffed peppers in shallow baking dish. Cover with foil and bake until heated through, about 20 to 25 minutes.

GRILLED WILD SALMON WITH PESTO

Serves 2

Two 6-ounce salmon filets
1 teaspoon extra-virgin
   olive oil
1 bunch spinach

2 teaspoons butter,
   clarified
Basil Pesto (see recipe,
   page 198)

Preheat oven to 350°F. Brush salmon filets with olive oil on both sides. Place skin side down in baking dish. Bake 6 to 8 minutes or until center of fish is opaque.

In pot, melt butter over medium heat. Add spinach and cover to steam, about 1 to 2 minutes. Remove from heat, plate spinach, and top with salmon.

SWEET POTATO–CRUSTED WILD SALMON

Serves 2

1 teaspoon coconut oil
Two 6-ounce wild Alaskan
   salmon filets

1 large egg, beaten
1 large sweet potato,
   shredded

Preheat broiler. Oil baking dish with coconut oil. Brush beaten egg on top of salmon. Top salmon with shredded sweet potato. Arrange salmon on baking sheet and place in broiler at medium-high heat. Broil until salmon is opaque in middle when pierced with knife and potatoes are golden brown, about 6 to 10 minutes. Do not overcook salmon.

CAJUN CATFISH, MASHED PARSNIPS AND APPLES, AND ROASTED BRUSSELS SPROUTS

Serves 4

Roasted Brussels Sprouts (see Roasting Those Vegetables, page 121)

Mashed Parsnips and Apples

3 medium apples, cored, seeded, and chopped (can also substitute pears)
4 medium parsnips, peeled and chopped
¼ cup water

¼ cup unsweetend coconut milk
¼ teaspoon ground cinnamon
Sea salt and ground black pepper to taste

Combine apples, parsnips, and water in small pot. Bring to a boil and cook until parsnips are soft, about 20 minutes. Remove from heat and drain any liquid. Place mixture in food processor or blender and add the coconut milk and cinnamon. Blend until pureed. Return to pot to reheat over low heat. Season with salt and pepper before serving.

Cajun Catfish

Four 6-ounce catfish filets
¼ cup fresh lemon juice

2 tablespoons Cajun seasonings

Preheat oven to 350°F. Arrange fish in single layer in baking dish. Sprinkle lemon juice on fish and then pat on Cajun seasoning. Bake 10 to 12 minutes or until fish is lightly browned.

ALMOND-CRUSTED TILAPIA AND
SWEET POTATO MASH

Serves 2

1 large egg

2 teaspoons unsweetened
  almond milk

1 cup almond meal

¼ teaspoon sea salt

¼ teaspoon ground black
  pepper

½ teaspoon onion powder

½ teaspoon garlic powder

1 tablespoon parsley,
  chopped

Two 6-ounce tilapia filets

1 teaspoon coconut oil

2 medium sweet potatoes,
  peeled and cut into
  small pieces

1 tablespoon butter

¼ cup coconut milk

¼ teaspoon ground
  cinnamon

Preheat oven to 400°F. In shallow bowl, beat egg and almond milk and set aside. Combine almond meal, salt, pepper, onion and garlic powder, and chopped parsley in another shallow bowl. Dip tilapia filets into egg mixture and then into almond mixture to coat well. Arrange fish in shallow baking dish coated lightly with coconut oil. Bake 8 to 10 minutes or until lightly browned.

Boil sweet potatoes until they are tender, about 20 to 30 minutes. Drain potatoes and mash them with a fork or potato masher. Add in butter, coconut milk, and cinnamon until well blended together.

FISH TACOS

Serves 4

Four 4-ounce pieces
  white fish (such as
  mahimahi, tilapia, or
  flounder)
2 limes
1 teaspoon chili powder
1 tablespoon coconut oil

½ cup cabbage, shredded
1 teaspoon cilantro,
  chopped
1 cup salsa
8 large romaine lettuce
  leaves

Marinate fish in juice of 1 lime and chili powder for 15 minutes. Heat coconut oil in large skillet. Add fish and cook until center of fish becomes opaque. Flake cooked fish and shredded cabbage inside large romaine leaves. Top with fresh squeezed lime juice, cilantro, and salsa; roll up lettuce leaf like a wrap and serve.

SESAME SEARED TUNA WITH SEAWEED SALAD

Serves 2

Sesame Seared Tuna

Two 6-ounce ahi tuna
  steaks
½ teaspoon sea salt

½ teaspoon ground black
  pepper
1 tablespoon sesame oil
1 teaspoon sesame seeds

Heat skillet on medium-high heat. Rinse and pat dry tuna steaks. Sprinkle with salt and pepper. Brush both sides of tuna steak with sesame oil and coat with sesame seeds.

Sear steaks, cooking 2 to 3 minutes per side for rare, 4 to 5 minutes per side for well done.

Seaweed Salad

2 ounces dried wakame
seaweed
⅓ cup rice vinegar

1 teaspoon sesame oil
4 tablespoons sesame
seeds, toasted

Place wakame seaweed in mixing bowl filled with water and soak for 20 to 30 minutes. Remove from water and squeeze dry. Cut into thin strips and place in large bowl. In separate bowl, whisk together vinegar and oil. Pour over seaweed and top with sesame seeds; toss well and serve.

COCONUT SHRIMP WITH SESAME BOK CHOY

Serves 2

½ cup coconut milk
½ cup shredded coconut
8 large shrimp, peeled and
deveined
1 tablespoon coconut oil
2 tablespoons sesame
seeds
2 teaspoons extra-virgin
olive oil

¼ cup onions, chopped
1 tablespoon garlic,
minced
4 stalks bok choy, torn or
cut into ½-inch-thick
pieces
Sea salt and ground black
pepper to taste

Place coconut milk and shredded coconut into two separate bowls. Dip shrimp into coconut milk bowl and then dip into coconut bowl to be sure whole shrimp is covered in coconut flakes. In small skillet, heat coconut oil to medium-high. Place in skillet and lightly brown both sides until shrimp is cooked, about 3 to 5 minutes.

Heat large skillet over medium heat. Add sesame seeds and cook until lightly toasted for about 1 to 2 minutes; place seeds in bowl and set aside. Add olive oil to same skillet and sauté onions until translucent. Add garlic and cook another minute. Add bok choy, salt, and pepper, and stir-fry over medium-high heat until bok choy is cooked, about 3 to 5 minutes. Sprinkle sesame seeds on top and toss. Remove from heat and serve.

GRILLED ROSEMARY-GARLIC SHRIMP WITH GRILLED VEGETABLES

Serves 2

Grilled Rosemary-Garlic Shrimp

2 garlic cloves, run through a garlic press
1 tablespoon fresh rosemary leaves, minced
¼ cup extra-virgin olive oil
Juice of 1 lemon

1 pound shrimp, peeled and deveined
Bamboo or metal skewers (if using bamboo, soak skewers in water for 30 minutes)

Combine garlic, rosemary, olive oil, and lemon juice. Add shrimp and marinate 1 hour. Skewer shrimp. Grill shrimp for 2 minutes per side at 400°F.

Grilled Vegetables

1 medium zucchini, halved lengthwise
1 medium eggplant, halved lengthwise

1 medium yellow pepper, halved	1 tablespoon extra-virgin olive oil
	1 teaspoon sea salt

Preheat grill or grill pan to 350°F. Place vegetables on cutting board and drizzle with olive oil and sprinkle with salt. Grill the zucchini and eggplant, turning often, until lightly charred and tender, about 10 to 12 minutes; the yellow pepper for 5 minutes.

CUCUMBER SUSHI* AND WASABI MASHED "POTATOES"

Serves 4

Wasabi Mashed "Potatoes"

1 head cauliflower, torn into florets	1 tablespoon chives, minced
½ cup unsweetened coconut milk or almond milk	1 tablespoon butter
	½ teaspoon sea salt
1 teaspoon wasabi powder	Ground black pepper to taste

In pot, steam cauliflower in 2 cups water until fork tender, about 20 to 25 minutes. Transfer cauliflower and any remaining liquid to blender or food processor and blend until smooth. Heat milk in small saucepan over medium heat for 5 minutes. Whisk in wasabi powder until dissolved. Add milk mixture, chives, butter, salt, and pepper to cauliflower. Mix well to combine; serve immediately.

---

* You can find sushi wrapped in cucumber without rice at Japanese restaurants and some supermarkets.

SNACKS

Chicken-Vegetable Soup

Bacon-Wrapped Dates

Paleo Dip with Vegetables

Crabmeat-Cucumber Salad

Crabmeat-Stuffed Mushrooms

California Chicken Salad

Avocado Turkey Boat

Smoked Salmon and Red Pepper Roll-Ups

Ants on a Log

Chicken, Avocado, and Walnut Salad

Watermelon, Avocado, and Hearts of Palm Salad

Smoked Salmon, Fennel, and Dill Salad

Grilled Shrimp Skewers

Mojito Shrimp Salad

Shrimp Ceviche

Gazpacho

Salmon Salad

Tuna Salad

Turkey Pepper Open-Faced Sandwich

Deviled Guacamole Eggs

Apple Chips

Trail Mix

Chicken-Endive Boat

Turkey Avocado Roll-Ups

Gorgeous Coconut Protein Bars

Gorgeous Almond Protein Bars

Paleo Fruit Bars

CHICKEN-VEGETABLE SOUP

Although this is listed in the snack section, you can certainly use it as a meal!

Serves 4; each serving is 1 snack portion

Two 6-ounce skinless, boneless chicken breasts, chopped

6 cups water, broth, or chicken stock

5 carrots, cut into 2-inch pieces

2 onions, chopped

3 celery stalks, cut into 2-inch pieces

2 garlic cloves, minced

6 sprigs parsley, chopped

6 sprigs dill, chopped

1 bay leaf

1 teaspoon sea salt

¼ teaspoon ground black pepper

¼ cup parsley, chopped

Place all ingredients in large pot and bring to boil. Reduce heat and simmer, covered, until chicken is cooked through and vegetables are tender, about 45 minutes. Discard bay leaf before serving. (Soup may be divided into servings and frozen up to 1 month.)

Note: If you have bones from the chicken carcass on hand, throw them in the pot and cook with all the vegetables to boost the nutritional content.

BACON-WRAPPED DATES

2 slices pork bacon, cut in half

4 large dates, pitted

Wrap slice of bacon around pitted dates, place it on cooking sheet, and bake in oven for 20 to 25 minutes or until bacon is crispy. Let cool and serve.

PALEO DIP WITH VEGETABLES

1 head cauliflower
2 tablespoons extra-virgin olive oil
½ cup tahini
3 garlic cloves, minced

3 tablespoons fresh lemon juice
Sea salt and ground black pepper to taste

Cut up raw vegetables: cherry tomatoes, carrots, celery, bell peppers, cucumber, zucchini, and green beans.

Chop cauliflower and place in pot. Steam with 2 cups water until fork tender, about 20 minutes. Set aside to cool for 10 minutes. Place cauliflower in food processor with olive oil, tahini, garlic, lemon juice, sea salt, and pepper; blend until desired consistency. Serve with raw veggies. Refrigerates for up to 1 week.

CRABMEAT-CUCUMBER SALAD

1 cucumber, chopped

1 cup lump crabmeat, picked over

1 tablespoon grapeseed oil

2 tablespoons rice vinegar

2 large tomatoes, thickly sliced

In medium bowl, combine cucumber, crabmeat, oil, and vinegar. Arrange crabmeat salad atop tomato slices.

CRABMEAT-STUFFED MUSHROOMS

Serves 4

2 cups lump crabmeat (1 pound)

1 large egg

2 tablespoons fresh lemon juice

1 teaspoon Dijon mustard

Sea salt and ground black pepper to taste

24 medium mushrooms, such as button or cremini, stems removed

Preheat oven to 350°F. Mix together all ingredients, except mushrooms, in bowl. Place mushrooms faceup on baking sheet. Divide crab mixture among mushroom tops and bake 20 minutes.

CALIFORNIA CHICKEN SALAD

One 6-ounce grilled
chicken breast

2 cups fresh spinach,
rinsed

10 cherry tomatoes,
halved

1 rib celery, sliced into
¼-inch pieces

1 carrot, peeled and sliced
into ¼-inch pieces

1 tablespoon almonds,
toasted

¼ avocado

1 teaspoon olive oil

1 tablespoon balsamic
vinegar

Place chicken atop spinach with cherry tomatoes, celery, carrots, toasted almonds, and ¼ avocado. Drizzle olive oil and balsamic vinegar on top.

AVOCADO TURKEY BOAT

½ avocado, pit removed

2 ounces cooked turkey,
chopped into small
pieces

½ tomato, chopped

Mix turkey and tomato together in small bowl; place atop center avocado half.

SMOKED SALMON AND RED PEPPER ROLL-UPS

3 ounces smoked wild
Alaskan salmon, cut
into thin strips

1 red bell pepper, cut into
slices

Wrap pieces of salmon around pepper slices.

ANTS ON A LOG

2 tablespoons almond
butter

4 celery sticks
1 tablespoon raisins

Spoon ½ tablespoon almond butter on each celery stick and
sprinkle raisins on top.

CHICKEN, AVOCADO, AND WALNUT SALAD

2 ounces chicken,
shredded
¼ avocado, chopped
¼ cup walnuts

1 teaspoon apple cider
vinegar
Sea salt to taste

Mix together all ingredients in bowl and serve.

WATERMELON, AVOCADO, AND
HEARTS OF PALM SALAD

Serves 2

1 cup watermelon, diced
½ avocado, diced
½ cup hearts of palm, chopped, rinsed, and drained

½ cup almonds, slivered
3 tablespoons balsamic vinegar

Mix ingredients together in a medium bowl. Serve immediately.

SMOKED SALMON, FENNEL, AND DILL SALAD

3 ounces sliced wild smoked salmon, chopped
1 medium fennel bulb, chopped
1 medium shallot, minced
8 Kalamata olives, chopped

½ medium cucumber, peeled, seeded, and chopped
1 tablespoon capers, drained
1 tablespoon dill, chopped
1 teaspoon fresh lemon juice

Place all ingredients in bowl, toss, and serve.

GRILLED SHRIMP SKEWERS

Serves 2

8 shrimp, shelled and
deveined
2 tablespoons extra-virgin
olive oil
1 tablespoon ground
cumin
1 tablespoon curry powder
1 teaspoon ground black
pepper

8 cherry tomatoes
½ red onion, chopped into
2-inch pieces
Bamboo or metal skewers
(if using bamboo, soak
skewers in water for
30 minutes)

Preheat grill pan. Place shrimp in medium-sized bowl and toss with olive oil, cumin, curry powder and black pepper to coat thoroughly. Place shrimp on skewers, alternating with cherry tomatoes and onions. Cook for 2 to 3 minutes per side or until shrimp is pink in color.

MOJITO SHRIMP SALAD

1 cup cooked small
shrimp (approximately
6 ounces)
½ avocado, diced
2 teaspoons lime zest

2 tablespoons fresh lime
juice
2 tablespoons mint leaves,
slivered

Mix together all ingredients in bowl and serve chilled.

SHRIMP CEVICHE

Serves 2

10 (about ⅓ pound) cooked shrimp, cut into pieces
2 tablespoons red onion, chopped
½ cup tomatoes, diced
½ cup fresh lime juice
½ cup fresh lemon juice
2 teaspoons cilantro, chopped

Combine all ingredients in small bowl. Let stand for 10 minutes and serve.

GAZPACHO

Serves 6

4 plum tomatoes, peeled and chopped
1 medium cucumber, peeled and chopped
1 green pepper, cored, seeded, and chopped
2 scallions, sliced
2 cups organic canned or fresh tomato juice
2 tablespoons fresh lemon juice
¼ teaspoon cayenne pepper
Fresh parsley (for garnish)

Place all ingredients in blender or food processor and mix together well. Chill in refrigerator at least 2 hours or overnight. Place in bowl and serve with fresh parsley as garnish.

SALMON SALAD

One 6-ounce can wild
  salmon
½ tomato, diced
¼ cup red onion, diced
1 teaspoon olive oil

2 teaspoons white
  balsamic vinegar
Garlic salt and ground
  black pepper to taste

Mix together all ingredients in bowl, toss, and serve.

TUNA SALAD

One 6-ounce can tuna
  fish
½ cup celery, diced
1 tablespoon extra-virgin
  olive oil

1 tablespoon apple cider
  vinegar
1 teaspoon parsley,
  chopped
1 tomato, thinly sliced

In bowl, mix together all ingredients except tomato slices.
Spoon mixture on top of tomato slices and serve.

TURKEY PEPPER OPEN-FACED SANDWICH

1 bell pepper (red, orange,
  or yellow)
2 tablespoons mustard or
  guacamole

4 ounces sliced turkey
  breast

Slice pepper in half; remove stem and seeds. Divide 2 tablespoons mustard or guacamole between both pepper halves.

Divide 4 ounces sliced turkey breast between both pepper halves and enjoy.

DEVILED GUACAMOLE EGGS

2 large eggs, hard boiled
1 lime, juiced
1 teaspoon fresh cilantro, chopped

⅛ teaspoon cayenne powder
½ avocado

Cut hard-boiled eggs in half lengthwise and scoop out yolk. Place yolks, lime juice, cilantro, and cayenne in bowl and mash together with a large fork. Split avocado in half and remove pit; scoop meat out with large spoon and mash in with egg yolk mixture. Spoon egg yolk mixture back into center of each egg white, and serve immediately or store in airtight container in fridge. Will keep up to 48 hours.

APPLE CHIPS

3 apples, thinly sliced and cored

2 tablespoons ground cinnamon

Preheat oven to 250°F. Line a baking sheet with parchment paper. Place apple slices on baking sheets and sprinkle with cinnamon. Bake until apples are dry and crisp, about 1½ to 2 hours, flipping the apples after 1 hour. Cool and serve. Apple chips are best eaten on the day they are made, but they will keep fresh in an airtight container for up to a week.

TRAIL MIX

Makes 2 cups

½ cup almonds
½ cup cashews
¼ cup sunflower seeds

¼ cup pumpkin seeds
¼ cup dried cranberries
¼ cup raisins

Put all ingredients in plastic bag and shake it well to mix. Store in freezer for optimal freshness. One serving equals ½ cup.

CHICKEN-ENDIVE BOAT

1 cup chicken, cooked and shredded
10 sliced cherry tomatoes
¼ cup red onion, diced

5 endive leaves
Sea salt and ground black pepper to taste

Divide chicken, tomatoes, and onion among endive leaves. Season to taste and enjoy.

TURKEY AVOCADO ROLL-UPS

3 slices turkey
¼ avocado, diced

Divide ¼ sliced avocado among 3 slices turkey. Roll up before eating.

GORGEOUS COCONUT PROTEIN BARS

Serves 3

½ cup vanilla whey protein powder

¼ cup coconut flour

¼ cup shredded coconut

¼ cup coconut milk

1 ounce dark chocolate, melted

Mix protein powder, coconut flour, and shredded coconut in bowl. Slowly add milk to make batter. (If mix is too watery, you can add more coconut flour.) After reaching desired consistency, divide mixture into 3 squares. Melt chocolate in bowl over a pot of water on low heat. Dip bars into chocolate and place in freezer for 30 minutes. Store in airtight container in fridge.

GORGEOUS ALMOND PROTEIN BARS

Serves 3

½ cup chocolate whey protein powder

¼ cup almond milk

¼ cup coconut flour

¼ cup almond flour

1 ounce dark chocolate, melted

Mix protein powder and coconut and almond flour in bowl. Slowly add milk to make batter. (If mix is too watery, you can add more coconut and almond flour.) After reaching desired consistency, divide mixture into 3 squares. Melt chocolate in bowl over a pot of water on low heat. Dip bars into chocolate and place in freezer for 30 minutes. Store in airtight container in fridge until ready for consumption.

PALEO FRUIT BARS

Makes 16 bars

2 cups dates, pitted
1 cup nuts, such as
    almonds, cashews, or
    pecans

1 cup dried cranberries

Place all ingredients in food processor and blend until mixed thoroughly. Pour mixture into an 8 x 8-inch pan and evenly press across bottom of pan. Refrigerate until set and then cut into bars. Store in airtight container in refrigerator.

Recommended Products
for Personal Use

Deodorants

Armpit Candy	www.armpitcandy.com
Aubrey Organics	www.aubrey-organics.com
Lafes	www.lafes.com
Misessence	www.amazon.com
Weleda	www.usa.weleda.com

Cosmetics and Skin Care

Acure Organics	www.acureorganics.com
Afterglow Cosmetics	www.afterglowcosmetics.com
Arbonne	www.arbonne.com
Ava Anderson	www.avaandersonnontoxic.com
Josie Maran Cosmetics	www.josiemarancosmetics.com
MakeupMakeup	www.makeupmakeup.com
Phyt's	www.phyts-usa.com
Relevé Organic Skincare	www.livinggorgeous.myemeraldstore.com
Suki	www.sukiskincare.com
Tata Harper	www.tataharperskincare.com

Sunscreens

www.ewg.org/2013sunscreen/
The Environmental Working Group is the nation's leading
environmental health research and advocacy organization. They
ensure that food and consumer products are free of harmful
chemicals.

Cell Phone Cases

Pong Research Corporation   www.pongresearch.com

Food and Supplements

Raw Coconut Aminos
    Coconut Secret   *www.coconutsecret.com*
Jerky
    Steve's Paleogoods   *www.stevespaleogoods.com*
Powdered Green Drinks
    PaleoGreens by
    Designs for Health   www.designsforhealth.com
Raw Milk
    A Campaign for Real Milk   www.real-milk.com
Whey Protein
    Action Whey   livinggorgeous
                                 .myemeraldstore.com

Wild Alaskan Salmon   www.vitalchoice.com
Wild Game, Meats, and Raw Milk   www.eatwild.com

Recommended Household Products

| Cleaning Products | www.ewg.org/guides/cleaners/content /top_products |
| Laundry Detergents | www.ewg.org/guides/categories/9-Laundry |

Acknowledgments

My heartfelt thanks go to the following people:

Celeste Fine, my sexy, fierce, amazing agent provocateur. The thousands of steps we have taken together on our collaborative journey humble me. You have always had my best interests at heart and have seen possibilities in me I never even saw in myself. Your talents are a gift, and I thank my lucky stars that I have you in my life.

The team at Gallery Books: Jeremie Ruby-Strauss, for projecting this book out to the universe and then letting me fulfill that dream—in spite of my salacious sense of humor; Emilia Pisani, for graciously weighing in with your thoughtful edits; Philip Bashe, for your extraordinary attention to detail in the copyedits; Kristin Dwyer, for rocking my publicity launch; Lisa Litwack, for your gorgeous cover design. You all raised the Paleo bar, and I am so proud of what we achieved together.

Harriet Bell, for your editorial guidance.

Sabrina Sarabella, my gorgeous intern, for helping me gather research and recipes.

Rachel Guy, for submitting photos and protocols for the exercise chapter. You are beautiful from the inside out, and I look forward to future collaborations.

My dear colleagues for generously sharing information and providing a source of support, encouragement, and inspiration:

Jade Teta, Jill Coleman, Charles Poliquin, Mark Houston, Jillian Sarno Teta, Jeannette Bessinger, Kaayla Daniel, Jeffrey Smith, Jonny Bowden, JJ Virgin, Mark Diaz, Debra Duby, Jason Boehm, Mark Schauss, David Zyla, Paula Owens, Deanna Minich, and Dan Katz.

The staff at Saugatuck Craft Butchery, for rounding out my knowledge on pastured meats.

Nicole Paul, Brian Delaney, Sandi Silk, and Melanie DeGreling, Kathryn Herrington, Judy Weiss, Jodi Greenspan, Michele Blumberg, and Judy Bowman. I love you madly and thank you from the depths of my heart for so many years of deep, soulful friendships. The Connecticut Whores: Dina Rutig, Caroline Covert, Karen Buchichio, Michele Olbrys, and Brian Buchichio (our honorary whore). Andrea Davis and Jen Siegel. I love you and am so grateful for all the love, laughter, joy, and sanity you bring into my life.

Eileen, Lina, Lynda, and Nora: thank you for selflessly sharing your most personal stories with me about what life was like after going Paleo. Your kindness and generosity are deeply appreciated.

All the readers, family, and friends who continue to support my books and spread the gorgeous word. Your patronage and viral marketing are a driving force behind my brand.

Lastly, huge piles of love for my team at home, Jeremy and Benjamin. I would never be where I am today without your love and support. And Ben, I will never tire of hearing you tell me I'll be famous one day.

Bibliography

Abboud, Leila. "Expect a Food Fight as U.S. Sets to Revise Diet Guidelines." *Wall Street Journal*, August 8, 2003, B1.

Agrawal, R., and F. Gomez-Pinilla. "'Metabolic Syndrome' in the Brain: Deficiency in Omega-3 Fatty Acid Exacerbates Dysfunctions in Insulin Receptor Signalling and Cognition." *Journal of Physiology* 590, pt. 10 (May 1, 2012): 2485–99.

Alleva, E., and J. Brock. "Statement from the Work Session on Environmental Endocrine-Disrupting Chemicals: Neural, Endocrine, and Behavioral Effects: The Problem." *Toxicology and Industrial Health* 14, nos. 1–2 (January 1998): 1–8.

Allsop, K. A., and J. B. Miller. "Honey Revisited: A Reappraisal of Honey in Preindustrial Diets." *British Journal of Nutrition* 75, no. 4 (April 1996): 513–20.

Aris A., and S. Leblanc. "Maternal and fetal exposure to pesticides associated to genetically modified foods in Eastern Townships of Quebec, Canada." *Reproductive Toxicology* 31 (2011): 528–33.

Avena, N. M., P. Rada, and B. G. Hoebel. "Sugar and Fat Bingeing Have Notable Differences in Addictive-like Behavior." *Journal of Nutrition* 139, no. 3 (March 2009): 623–28.

Baillie-Hamilton, P. F. "Chemical Toxins: A Hypothesis to Explain the Global Obesity Epidemic." *Journal of Alternative and Complementary Medicine* 8, no. 2 (April 2002): 185–92.

Benson, J. "'Monsanto Protection Act' to grant biotech industry total immunity over GM crops?" *Natural News*, Sunday, July 15, 2012.

Berry, I. "Syngenta Settles Weedkiller Lawsuit." *Wall Street Journal*, May 25, 2012.

Burns, CM. "Higher serum glucose levels are associated with cerebral hypometabolism in Alzheimer regions." *Neurology*, 2013 April 23; 80(17): 1557–64.

Broussard, J. L., D. A. Ehrmann, E. Van Cauter, E. Tasali, and M. J. Brady. "Impaired Insulin Signaling in Human Adipocytes After Experimental Sleep Restriction: A Randomized, Crossover Study." *Annals of Internal Medicine* 157, no. 8 (October 16, 2012): 549–57.

Carman, J. A., et al. A long-term toxicology study on pigs fed a combined genetically modified (GM) soy and GM maize diet. *Journal of Organic Systems* 8(1)(2013).

Centers for Disease Control and Prevention. "Fourth National Report on Human Exposure to Environmental Chemicals." NCEH Publication No. 03-0022. Atlanta: Centers for Disease Control.

Dadd, Debra Lynn. *Home Safe Home: Protecting Yourself and Your Family from Everyday Toxics and Harmful Household Products*. New York: Jeremy P. Tarcher/Putnam, 1997.

DeGrassi, A. "Genetically modified crops and sustainable poverty alleviation in sub-Saharan Africa: An assessment of current evidence." Third World Network–Africa, June 2003.

Dhiman, T. R., G. R. Anand, L. D. Satter, and M. W. Pariza. "Conjugated Linoleic Acid Content of Milk from Cows Fed Different Diets." *Journal of Dairy Science* 82, no. 10 (October 1999): 2146–56.

Dolecek, T. A., and G. Granditis. "Dietary Polyunsaturated Fatty Acids and Mortality in the Multiple Risk Factor Intervention Trial (MRFIT)." *World Review of Nutrition and Dietetics* 66 (1991): 205–16.

Duckett, S. K., D. G. Wagner, L. D. Yates, H. G. Dolezal, and S. G. May. "Effects of Time on Feed on Beef Nutrient Composition." *Journal of Animal Science* 71, no. 8 (August 1993): 2079–88.

Duckett, S. K., J. P. Neel, J. P. Fontenot, and W. M. Clapham. "Effects of Winter Stocker Growth Rate and Finishing System on: III. Tissue Proximate, Fatty Acid, Vitamin and Cholesterol Content." *Journal of Animal Science* 87, no. 9 (September 2009): 2961–70.

Fallon, Sally and Mary Enig. *Nourishing Traditions: The Cookbook that Challenges Politically Correct Nutrition and the Diet Dictocrats.* Washington, DC: Newtrends Publishing, Inc.; Revised and Updated 2nd edition, October 1, 1999.

Farnsworth, E., N. D. Luscombe, M. Noakes, G. Wittert, E. Argyiou, and P. M. Clifton. "Effect of a High-Protein, Energy-Restricted Diet on Body Composition, Glycemic Control, and Lipid Concentrations in Overweight and Obese Hyperinsulinemic Men and Women." *American Journal of Clinical Nutrition* 78, no. 1 (July 2003): 31–39.

Forsythe, C. E., S. D. Phinney, M. L. Fernandez, E. E. Quann, R. J. Wood, D. M. Bibus, W. J. Kraemer, et al. "Comparison of Low Fat and Low Carbohydrate Diets on Circulating Fatty Acid Composition and Markers of Inflammation." *Lipids* 43, no. 1 (January 2008): 65–77

Foster, G. D., H. R. Wyatt, J. O. Hill, B. G. McGuckin, C. Brill, B. S. Mohammed, P. O. Szapary, et al. "A Randomized Trial of a Low-Carbohydrate Diet for Obesity." *New England Journal of Medicine* 348, no. 21 (May 22, 2003): 2082–90.

Gathura, G. "GM technology fails local potatoes." *The Daily Nation* (Kenya), 29 January 2004.

Gavaler, J. S. "Alcoholic Beverages as a Source of Estrogens." *Alcohol Health & Research World* 22, no. 3 (1998): 220–27.

Gibson, S. A., C. McFarlan, S. Hay, and G. T. Macfarlane. "Significance of Microflora in Proteolysis in the Colon." *Applied and Environmental Microbiology* 55, no. 3 (March 1989): 679–83.

Gorski, Barbara L. "Pastured Poultry Products." Sustainable Agriculture Research & Education. (1999). http://mysare.sare.org/mySARE/assocfiles/915436Final.pdf.

Holtcamp, W. "Obesogens: An Environmental Link to Obesity." *Environmental Health Perspectives* 120, no. 2 (February 2012): a62–a68.

Ho, Mae-Wan. "GM Ban Long Overdue: Dozens Ill & Five Deaths in the Philippines." Institute of Science in Society press release (June 2, 2006). www.isis.org.uk/GMBanLongOverdue.php.

Ho, Mae-Wan, and Sam Burcher. "Cows Ate GM Maize & Died." Institute of Science in Society press release (January 13, 2004). www.isis.org.uk/CAGMMAD.php.

Hovinga, M. E., M. Sowers, and H. E. Humphrey. "Environmental Exposure and Lifestyle Predictors of Lead, Cadmium, PCB, and DDT Levels in Great Lakes Fish Eaters." *Archives of Environmental Health* 48, no. 2 (April–May 1993): 98–104.

Hyman, M. "Systems Biology, Toxins, Obesity, and Functional Medicine." *Alternative Therapies in Health and Medicine* 13, no. 2 (March–April 2007): S134–S139.

Imbeault, P., A. Tremblay, J. A. Simoneau, and D. R. Joanisse. "Weight Loss–Induced Rise in Plasma Pollutant Is Associated with Reduced Skeletal Muscle Oxidative Capacity." *American Journal of Physiology—Endocrinology and Metabolism* 282, no. 3 (March 2002): E574–E579.

Ip, C., J. A. Scimeca, and H. J. Thompson. "Conjugated Linoleic Acid: A Powerful Anticarcinogen from Animal Fat Sources." *Cancer* 74, supplement 3 (August 1994): 1050–54.

Klentzeris, L. D., J. N. Bulmer, T. C. Li, L. Morrison, A. Warren, and I.D. Cooke. "Lectin Binding of Endometrium in Women with Unexplained Infertility." *Fertility and Sterility* 56, no. 4 (October 1991): 660–67.

Knight, E. L., M. J. Stampfer, S. E. Hankinson, D. Spiegelman, and G. C. Curhan. "The Impact of Protein Intake on Renal Function Decline in Women with Normal Renal Function or Mild Renal Insufficiency." *Annals of Internal Medicine* 138, no. 6 (March 18, 2003): 460–67.

Layman, D. K., R. A. Boileau, D. J. Erickson, J. E. Painter, H. Shiue, C. Sather, and D. D. Christou. "A Reduced Ratio of Carbohydrate to Protein Improves Body Composition and Blood Lipid Profiles During Weight Loss in Adult Women." *Journal of Nutrition* 133, no. 2 (February 1, 2003): 411–17.

Layman, D. K., E. Evans, J. I. Baum, J. Seyler, D. J. Erickson, and R. A. Boileau. "Dietary Protein and Exercise Have Additive Effects on Body Composition During Weight Loss in Adult Women." *Journal of Nutrition* 135, no. 8 (August 1, 2005): 1903–10.

Leidy, H. J., R. J. Lepping, C. R. Savage, and C. T. Harris. "Neural Responses to Visual Food Stimuli After a Normal Vs. Higher Protein Breakfast in Breakfast-Skipping Teens: A Pilot fMRI Study." *Obesity* 19, no. 10 (October 2011): 2019–25.

Leidy, H. J., M. Tang, C. L. Armstrong, C. B. Martin, and W. W. Campbell. "The Effects of Consuming Frequent, Higher Protein Meals on Appetite and Satiety During Weight Loss in Overweight/Obese Men." *Obesity* 19, no. 4 (April 1, 2011): 818–24.

Lopez-Bote, C. J., R. Sanz Arias, A. I. Rey, A. Castano, B. Isabel, and J. Thos. "Effect of Free-Range Feeding on Omega-3 Fatty Acid and Alpha-Tocopherol Content and Oxidative Stability of Eggs." *Animal Feed Science and Technology* 72, no. 1 (May 1998): 33–40.

Lotan, R., and A. Raz. "Lectins in Cancer Cells." *Annals of the New York Academy of Sciences* 551 (December 1988): 385–96; discussion, 396–98.

Macfarlane, G. T., C. Allison, S. A. Gibson, and J. H. Cummings. "Contribution of the Microflora to Proteolysis in the Human Large Intestine." *Journal of Applied Microbiology* 64, no. 1 (January 1988): 37–46.

McAfee, A. J., E. M. McSorley, G. J. Cuskelly, A. M. Fearon, B. W. Moss, J. A. Beattie, J. M. Wallace, et al. "Red Meat from Animals Offered a Grass Diet Increases Plasma and Platelet *n*-3 PUFA in Healthy Consumers." *British Journal of Nutrition* 105, no. 1 (January 2011): 80–89.

Mortality in Sheep Flocks After Grazing on Bt Cotton Fields—Warangal District, Andhra Pradesh: Report of the Preliminary Assessment (April 2006). http://gmwatch.org/latest-listing/1-news-items/6416-mortality-in-sheep-flocks-after-grazing-on-bt-cotton-fields-warangal-district-andhra-pradesh-2942006%GM-Watch.

"Monsanto's showcase project in Africa fails." *New Scientist*, vol. 181, no. 2433, February 7, 2004.

Moreira, P. I. "High-sugar Diets, Type 2 Diabetes and Alzheimer's Disease." *Current Opinion in Clinical Nutrition & Metabolic Care*, no. 16(4)(July 2013): 440–5.

Mousa, N. A., R. Eiada, P. Crystal, D. Nayot, and R. F. Casper. "The Effect of Acute Aromatase Inhibition on Breast Parenchymal Enhancement in Magnetic Resonance Imaging: A Prospective Pilot Clinical Trial." *Menopause* 19, no. 4 (April 2012): 420–25.

Nedeltcheva, A. V., J. M. Kilkus, J. Imperial, D. A. Schoeller, and P. D. Penev. "Insufficient Sleep Undermines Dietary Efforts to Reduce Adiposity." *Annals of Internal Medicine* 153, no. 7 (October 5, 2010): 435–41.

Oski, Frank A., MD. *Don't Drink Your Milk! New Frightening Medical Facts About the World's Most Overrated Nutrient.* Ringgold, GA: TEACH Services, 1992.

Parker, B., M. Noakes, N. Luscombe, and P. Clifton. "Effect of a High-Protein, High-Monounsaturated Fat Weight Loss Diet on Glycemic Control and Lipid Levels in Type 2 Diabetes." *Diabetes Care* 25 (March 2002): 425–30.

Pearson, A. M., and T. R. Dutson, eds. *Growth Regulation in Farm Animals. Advances in Meat Research.* London: Elsevier Science Publishers Ltd, 1991, vol. 7.

Perkin, M. R. "Unpasteurized Milk: Health or Hazard?" *Clinical & Experimental Allergy* 37, no. 5 (May 2007): 627–30.

Perkin, M. R., and D. P. Strachan. "Which Aspects of the Farming Lifestyle Explain the Inverse Association with Childhood Allergy?" *Journal of Allergy and Clinical Immunology* 117, no. 6 (June 2006): 1374–81.

Pettifor, J. M., H. Stein, A. Herman, F. P. Ross, T. Blumenfeld, and G. P. Moodley. "Mineral Homeostasis in Very Low Birth Weight Infants Fed Either Own Mother's Milk or Pooled Pasteurized Preterm Milk." *Journal of Pediatric Gastroenterology and Nutrition* 5, no. 2 (March–April 1986): 248–53.

Ponte, P. I., S. P. Alves, R. J. Bessa, L. M. Ferreira, L. T. Gama, J. L. Brás, C. M. Fontes, et al. "Influence of Pasture Intake on the Fatty Acid Composition and Cholesterol, Tocopherols, and Tocotrienols Content in Meat from Free-Range Broilers." *Poultry Science* 87, no. 1 (January 2008): 80–88.

Ponte, P. I., J. A. Prates, J. P. Crespo, D. G. Crespo, J. L. Maorão, S. P. Alves, R. J. Bessa, et al. "Restricting the Intake of a Cereal-Based Feed in Free Range-Pastured Poultry: Effects on Performance and Meat Quality." *Poultry Science* 87, no. 10 (October 2008): 2032–42.

Prentice, R. L., B. Caan, R. T. Chlebowski, R. Patterson, L. H. Kuller, J. K. Ockene, K. L. Margolis, et al. "Low-Fat Dietary Pattern and Risk of Invasive Breast Cancer: The Women's Health Initiative Randomized Controlled Dietary Modification Trial." *Journal of the American Medical Association* 295, no. 6 (February 8, 2006): 629–42.

Ratliff, J., J. O. Leite, R. de Ogburn, M. J. Puglisi, J. VanHeest, and M. L. Fernandez. "Consuming Eggs for Breakfast Influences Plasma Glucose and Ghrelin, While Reducing Energy Intake During the Next 24 Hours in Adult Men." *Nutrition Research* 30, no. 2 (February 2010): 96–103.

Pusztai, A. "Can Science Give Us the Tools for Recognizing Possible Health Risks of GM Food?" *Nutrition and Health* 16, no. 2 (2002): 73–84.

Report of the Panel on Macronutrients, Subcommittees on Upper Reference Levels of Nutrients and Interpretation and Uses of Dietary Reference Intakes, and the Standing Committee on the Scientific Evaluation of Dietary Reference Intakes, Dietary reference Intakes for Energy, Carbohydrate, Fat, Fatty Acids, Cholesterol, Protein, and Amino Acids (macronutrients). National Academies Press (2005).

Riedler, J., C. Braun-Fahrländer, W. Eder, M. Schreuer, M. Waser, S. Maisch, D. Carr, et al. "Exposure to Farming in Early Life and Development of Asthma and Allergy: A Cross-sectional Survey." *Lancet* 358, no. 9288 (October 6, 2001): 1129–33.

Robinson, Jo. *Pasture Perfect: How You Can Benefit from Choosing Meat, Eggs, and Dairy Products from Grass-Fed Animals.* Vashon, WA: Vashon Island Press, 2004.

Santos, F. L., et al. "Systematic review and meta-analysis of clinical trials of the effects of low carbohydrate diets on cardiovascular risk factors." *Obesity Review* 13(11) (November 2012): 1048–66.

St-Onge, M. P., A. McReynolds, Z. B. Trivedi, A. L. Roberts, M. Sy, and J. Hirsch. "Sleep Restriction Leads to Increased Activation of Brain Regions Sensitive to Food Stimuli." *American Journal of Clinical Nutrition* 95, no. 4 (April 2012): 818–24.

Shai, I., D. Schwarzfuchs, Y. Henkin, D. R. Shahar, S. Witkow, I. Greenberg, R. Golan, et al. "Weight Loss with a Low-Carbohydrate, Mediterranean, or Low-Fat Diet." *New England Journal of Medicine* 359, no. 3 (July 17, 2008): 229–41.

Shoemaker, R. C., and D. E. House. "A Time-Series Study of Sick Building Syndrome: Chronic, Biotoxin-Associated Illness from Exposure to Water-Damaged Buildings." *Neurotoxicology and Teratology* 27, no. 1 (January–February 2005): 29–46.

Siri-Tarino, P. W., Q. Sun, F. B. Hu, and R. M. Krauss. "Saturated Fat, Carbohydrate, and Cardiovascular Disease." *American Journal of Clinical Nutrition* 91, no. 3 (March 2010): 502–9.

Skov, A. R., S. Toubro, J. Bülow, K. Krabbe, H. H. Parving, and A. Astrup. "Changes in Renal Function During Weight Loss Induced by High Vs. Low-Protein Low-Fat Diets in Overweight Subjects." *International Journal of Obesity* 23, no. 11 (November 1999): 1170–77.

Skov A. R., S. Toubro, B. Ronn, L. Holm, and A. Astrup. "Randomized Trial on Protein Versus Carbohydrate in *Ad Libitum* Fat Reduced Diet for the Treatment of Obesity." *International Journal of Obesity* 23, no. 5 (May 1999): 528–36.

Smith, Jeffrey M. *Genetic Roulette: The Documented Health Risks of Genetically Engineered Foods.* Fairfield, IA: Yes! Books, 2007.

Stanley, W. C., E. R. Dabkowski, R. F. Ribeiro Jr., and K. A. O'Connell. "Dietary Fat and Heart Failure: Moving from Lipotoxicity to Lipoprotection." *Circulation Research* 110, no. 5 (March 2, 2012): 764–76.

Stein, H., D. Cohen, A. A. Herman, J. Rissick, U. Ellis, K. Bolton, J. Pettifor, et al. "Pooled Pasteurized Breast Milk and Untreated Own Mother's Milk in the Feeding of Very Low Birth Weight Babies: A Randomized Controlled Trial." *Journal of Pediatric Gastroenterology and Nutrition* 5, no. 2 (March–April 1986): 242–47.

Stellman, S. D., M. Djordjevic, J. Muscat, M. Citron, A. White, M. Kemeny, and E. Busch. "Adipose and Serum Levels of Organochlorinated Pesticides and PCB Residues in Long Island Women: Association with Age and Body Mass" (SER abstract). *American Journal of Epidemiology* S21 (1997): 81.

Trankina, M. L., D. C. Beitz, and A. H. Trenkle. "Effects of In Vitro Ronnel on Metabolic Activity in Subcutaneous Adipose Tissue and Skeletal Muscle from Steers." *Journal of Animal Science* 60, no. 3 (March 1985): 652–58.

Tremblay, A., C. Pelletier, E. Doucet, and P. Imbeault. "Thermogenesis and Weight Loss in Obese Individuals: A Primary Association with Organochlorine Pollution." *International Journal of Obesity* 28, no. 7 (July 2004): 936–39.

U.S. Department of Agriculture, U.S. Department of Health and Human Services. *Dietary Guidelines for Americans 2010*, 7th Edition, U.S. Government Printing Office (December 2010; accessed September 7, 2011).

U.S. Department of Agriculture and U.S. Department of Health and Human Services. *Report of the Dietary Guidelines Advisory Committee on the Dietary Guidelines for Americans, 2010.* (June 15, 2010) Available at: http://www.cnpp.usda .gov/DGAs2010-DGACReport.htm.

United States Tariff Commission. *Synthetic Organic Chemicals.* U.S. Government Printing Office [various documents], 1918–94.

Vázquez, R. I., et al. "Bacillus thuringiensis Cry1Ac protoxin is a potent systemic and mucosal adjuvant." *Scandinavian Journal of Immunology* 49 (1999): 578–84.

V. Lobo, et al. "Free radicals, antioxidants and functional foods: Impact on human health." *The Pharmacogenomics Journal* 4, no. 8 (July–Dec 2010): 118–126.

Volek, J. S., M. L. Fernandez, R. D. Feinman, and S. D. Phinney. "Dietary Carbohydrate Restriction Induces a Unique Metabolic State Positively Affecting Atherogenic Dyslipidemia, Fatty Acid Partitioning, and Metabolic Syndrome." *Progress in Lipid Research* 47, no. 5 (September 2008): 307–18.

Volek, J. S., M. J. Sharman, D. M. Love, N. G. Avery, A. L. Gómez, T. P. Scheett, and W. J. Kraemer. "Body Composition and Hormonal Responses to a Carbohydrate-Restricted Diet." *Metabolism* 51, no. 7 (July 2002): 864–70.

Wolk, A., et al. "A prospective study of association of monounsaturated fat and other types of fat with risk of breast cancer." *Archives of Internal Medicine* 158, no. 1 (Jan 12, 1998): 41–5.

Yamagishi, K., et al. "Dietary intake of saturated fatty acids and mortality from cardiovascular disease in Japanese: the Japan Collaborative Cohort Study for Evaluation of Cancer Risk (JACC) Study." *American Journal of Clinical Nutrition* 92, no. 4 (October 2010): 759–65.

Yamagishi, S. I., D. Edelstein, X. L. Du, Y. Kaneda, M. Guzmán, and M. Brownlee. "Leptin Induces Mitochondrial Superoxide Production and Monocyte Chemoattractant Protein-1 Expression in Aortic Endothelial Cells by Increasing Fatty Acid Oxidation via Protein Kinase A." *Journal of Biological Chemistry* 276, no. 27 (July 6, 2001): 25,096–100.

Yen, J. T., J. A. Nienaber, W. G. Pond, and V. H. Varel. "Effect of Carbadox on Growth, Fasting Metabolism, Thryroid Function and Gastrointestinal Tract in Young Pigs." *Journal of Nutrition* 115, no. 8 (August 1985): 970–79.

Zeisel S. H, K. A. da Costa. "Choline: an essential nutrient for public health." *Nutrition Reviews* 67, no. 11 (November 2009): 615–23.

Index